DICTIONARY
OF
PUBLIC
HEALTH
PROMOTION
AND
EDUCATION

DICTIONARY
OF
PUBLIC
HEALTH
PROMOTION
AND
EDUCATION
TERMS AND CONCEPTS

NAOMI N. MODESTE

SAGE Publications
International Educational and Professional Publisher
Thousand Oaks London New Delhi

For information address:

SAGE Publications, Inc.
2455 Teller Road
Thousand Oaks, California 91320
E-mail: order@sagepub.com

SAGE Publications Ltd.
6 Bonhill Street
London EC2A 4PU
United Kingdom

SAGE Publications India Pvt. Ltd.
M-32 Market
Greater Kailash I
New Delhi 110 048 India

Printed in the United States of America

Library of Congress Cataloging-in-Publication Data

Modeste, Naomi N.
    Dictionary of public health promotion and education: Terms and concepts / Naomi N. Modeste.
        p.   cm.
    Includes bibliographical references.
    ISBN 0-7619-0002-0 (cloth: alk. paper). — ISBN 0-7619-0003-9 (pbk.: alk. paper)
    1. Health education—Dictionaries. 2. Health promotion—Dictionaries. 3. Health education—Societies, etc.—Directories. 4. Health promotion—Societies, etc.—Directories. I. Title.
RA440.5.M634   1995
613'.03—dc20   95-35417

This book is printed on acid-free paper.

96 97 98 99 10 9 8 7 6 5 4 3 2 1

Sage Production Editor: Diane S. Foster

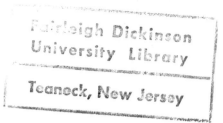
Contents

Foreword   vii
  by *Helen Hopp, Ph.D.*

Acknowledgments   ix

Introduction   xi

Part One: Dictionary of Terms and Concepts

     A   3

     B   7

     C   12

     D   28

     E   31

     F   38

     G   41

     H   44

     I   64

     L   70

     M   76

     N   80

     O   82

P   84

Q   96

R   99

S   102

T   114

U   117

V   118

W   120

Part Two:

Health and Professional Organizations   125

References   139

Suggested Readings   151

About the Author   161

Foreword

THIS guide of terms and concepts was prepared for health professionals in the field of health promotion and education, and for those in other professions that relate to health education. It covers a wide range of concepts commonly used by health educators, although it is not an exhaustive list of terms encountered by health professionals. In particular, the terms reflect the *process* of health promotion and education rather than focusing on disease-specific terminology. Key terms used in related public health disciplines, such as epidemiology, health administration, biostatistics, environmental health, and behavioral sciences, are also included, as most health educators must be familiar with these areas in their practice. Terms relevant to the four settings of health promotion and education (community, workplace, primary care, and school) are emphasized.

This guide was prompted by our graduate students' request for a reference list of terms that they could understand and employ consistently in their professional reading and writing. Additional contact with other health educators confirmed the need for such a guide.

Although it is impossible to present definitions that everyone will agree with, every attempt was made to cross-reference terms with a wide variety of key sources in health education. The references cited in the text and listed at the end of this guide were used as resource materials for deciding on definitions. Suggested Readings follow the References.

It is hoped that this guide will be useful to professionals in health promotion and education and their colleagues.

Helen Hopp, Ph.D.
School of Public Health
Loma Linda University

Acknowledgments

THIS book grew out of concerns shared by a number of my graduate students for a list of terms that can be used as a quick reference guide. The report of the 1990 Joint Committee on Health Education Terminology provided additional motivation for this work.

There are some individuals who deserve to be recognized here. Helen Hopp, a colleague in the department of health promotion and education, wrote the foreword, shared resources, and gave valuable assistance with several of the entries.

Christine Neish, Chairperson for the Department of Health Promotion and Education, and Joyce Hopp, Dean of the School of Allied Health Professions, provided administrative support and a critical review of the first draft.

Brick Lancaster, Associate Director for Health Education Practice and Policy at the Centers for Disease Control and Prevention; and Beverly Bradley, school health consultant, gave suggestions of terms and references that should be included or not included.

The help of all those who reviewed the manuscript and made suggestions and corrections, particularly the Sage reviewers, Brick Lancaster, Beverly Bradley, Noreen Clark, and Lawrence Green, is acknowledged here. Finally, recognition goes out to Christine Smedley, editor at Sage, for providing valuable suggestions, encouragement, and support throughout the process of this project. I take responsibility for any remaining weaknesses or omissions.

Introduction

THIS dictionary provides definitions of terms and concepts frequently used in public health promotion and education, written in a manner that can be easily comprehended. We in the field have learned a great deal about significant health-related concepts, but use terminology that is not necessarily found in any one text. This is an attempt to bring together a number of these terms under one cover for easy access.

The criterion for including terms and concepts was to select those that are widely used by a large number of people in the disciplines of public health, particularly health promotion and education. The intent was also to include terms in related disciplines with which health educators need to become familiar.

Many books and journal articles have been used as resources to select a wide range of terms and bring them together in dictionary form. The objective is that those who use this guide, whether student or professional, will be able to look up a definition without wading through scores of pages of books and articles. However, no attempt was made to include all of the terms and concepts ordinarily used, so this work is by no means exhaustive. It was not an easy task to select which resources to include as references and which to omit, as the same terms were referenced by many authors. Some important references may have been unintentionally omitted.

The definitions vary in length, as is to be expected given that some terms are simpler and more easily defined, whereas others call for a more detailed definition and even examples. Many of the entries have been cross-referenced to show how they relate to one another.

Some terms and concepts might not meet strict public health, health promotion, and health education definitions, but the reader should keep in mind that health education relies on many other disciplines, including epidemiology, biostatistics, theories of learning, and behavioral sciences.

This dictionary can be used as a companion to health education texts and courses of study by both undergraduate and graduate students. It can also serve as a source of reference for practicing health educators, faculty, and other health professionals involved in health promotion and education.

The dictionary is divided into two parts. Part One lists the selected terms alphabetically. This style was chosen because it provides a simple way of finding the entries and corresponds with most dictionary styles. If you wish to look up "Gannt chart," for example, go to "G" and find "Gannt chart." If you want to find a definition for "comprehensive health education," then go to "C" and look for it alphabetically. Do not become frustrated if a term you are searching for is not included; as stated previously, it is not the purpose of this dictionary to include all the terms and concepts appropriate to health promotion and education.

Part Two lists in alphabetical order some of the professional and voluntary agencies and organizations of which students and practicing health educators need to be aware. Like the list of terms, this section is not exhaustive. Key institutions are listed, including addresses where further information can be acquired.

A major objective in compiling this book was to keep it financially accessible to students, while at the same time including sufficient terminology and concepts to improve health education and promote literacy.

PART ONE

Dictionary of Terms and Concepts

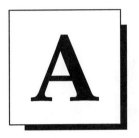

Abstinence

Abstinence is refraining from the use of drugs, alcohol, tobacco, and other substances or habits that tend to harm the body. Abstinence may also refer to refusing to engage in sex behaviors that may put individuals at risk for disease or disability.

Abstinence Violation Effect (AVE)

Abstinence violation effect (AVE), part of Marlatt and Gordon's model of the relapse process, involves a cognitive-emotional reaction that includes (a) guilt from relapsing and engaging in an undesired behavior (e.g., smoking) after quitting or changing the behavior (e.g., smoking cessation), which is discrepant from the new self-image (e.g., a nonsmoker); and (b) an attribution that the relapse episode was due to personal weakness. This usually results in perceptions of decreased self-efficacy in considering readopting a desired health behavior (Curry, Marlatt, & Gordon, 1987).

See **Relapse Prevention.**

A

Access to Health Care

Access to health care is the degree of ease with which individuals or groups of people obtain health care provided in a given community. Health educators look at access to health care in terms of transportation; location of facility; hours of operation; cost and financing (including health insurance); and social, ethnic, language, and geographic concerns that may help or hinder individuals in obtaining health care.

Administrative Diagnosis

An administrative diagnosis is an analysis of prevailing policies, resources, and circumstances in communities or organizations that help or hinder the development of a health promotion and education program.

The administrative diagnosis is included as part of the PRECEDE/ PROCEED Model (*see* PRECEDE/PROCEED Model) of health promotion planning and is important in funding decisions for a program. Administrative diagnosis includes resource assessment, setting time-table for activities, and budgeting (Green & Kreuter, 1991). The administrative diagnosis focuses on the assignment of the resources and responsibilities to implement and evaluate the proposed program or project.

Affective Domain

Affective domain is a category for classifying learning objectives that emphasize feeling and emotion, from the simplest outcomes to the most complex: personal interests, attitudes, values, appreciation, and methods of adjustment. Knowledge is more effective in shaping health-related behavior when combined with affective associations (Butler, 1994).

Example (a learning objective stated in the affective domain): By the end of this session, the student will be able to verbalize personal feelings about taking medication for hypertension.

Affective Learning

Affective learning is associated with beliefs, self-worth, appreciations, and values whereby learners are emotionally and actively involved in a learning experience and in relating to others. It can be opposed to cognitive learning (Himsl & Lambert, 1993).

See **Affective Domain** and **Cognitive Domain.**

A

Agent

An agent is an organism or object that transmits disease from the environment to the host or from one person to another. The agent acts with host and environmental characteristics to specify disease cases within a population (Friedman, 1980).

The term *agent* should not be limited to etiological agents. In health education and promotion the concept may include persons such as village and community health workers, community elders, teachers, and health educators who communicate health messages or act as channels through which ideas and innovations are transmitted to potential consumers.

Examples:

1. The human immunodeficiency virus (HIV), which causes acquired immunodeficiency syndrome (AIDS).
2. The tick that carries the virus for Colorado tick fever.
3. The mosquito (female anopheline) that carries the infection for malaria.

See **Host.**

Alma Ata Declaration

The Alma Ata Declaration was made by the World Health Assembly at the International Conference of Primary Health Care that met at Alma Ata, in the former Soviet Union, September 12, 1978.

The aim of this declaration was to commit all member countries of the World Health Organization (WHO) to the inclusion of lifestyle and behavioral factors and improvement of the environment within the principles of health for all by the year 2000. Primary health care was the principal thrust of the declaration, but it also incorporated community participation in an effort to protect and promote the health of all the people of the world (Bunton & Macdonald, 1992). The declaration was affirmed that health is a fundamental human right that should be made attainable for all people.

At-Risk Groups

At-risk groups are groups, or populations, who due to certain common existing economic, social, and environmental factors or behavioral characteristics may be prone to a certain disease or condition.

Examples:
Coal miners or coal workers
Parenteral drug users
Homosexuals and heterosexuals with multiple partners
Employees in a clinical laboratory
Persons practicing anal intercourse

Attitudes

Attitudes are favorable or unfavorable evaluative reactions or dispositions toward something, a situation, a person, or a group, exhibited in one's beliefs, feelings, or intended behavior (Fishbein & Ajzen, 1975; Pratkanis, Breckler, & Greenwald, 1989; Rajecki, 1990). An attitude that a person holds toward hypertension, for example, will help to guide or influence behavior intentions with respect to the problem.

Example: I (dis)like high-fat foods.

Since attitudes may be either positive or negative, there are times when helping people to change attitudes is as important as helping them to change behavior.

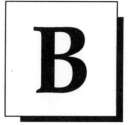

Behavior

A behavior is any observable response of a person to a stimulus or an action that has a "specific frequency, duration and purpose, whether conscious or unconscious" (Green & Kreuter, 1991, p. 429). Internal responses such as thinking or feeling may be inferred from observable behavior.

Behavior may also refer to how people react with one another as well as their environment and can be considered as a product of heredity, culture, and environment.

Example: Mothers in a given community breast-feed their babies from birth through the first 6 months without introducing other foods and liquids.

Behavior Modification

Behavior modification is one of the major approaches to learning and behavior change in health education. It is based on principles of respondent and operant learning involving changing an individual's response by manipulating the environment, specifically antecedent stimuli to, and reinforcement of, a behavior. Behavior modification may also be considered a coping strategy.

Behavior modification uses the following approach:

1. Identify the problem.
2. Describe the problem in behavioral terms.
3. Select target behaviors that are measurable.
4. Identify antecedents and consequences of the behavior.
5. Formulate behavioral objectives.
6. Devise and implement a behavioral change program.
7. Plan and execute an evaluation program. (Martin & Pear, 1992)

Example: Using the behavior modification approach to reduce overeating would involve the following steps. First, specify the behavioral goal(s): Reducing the number of snacks or amount of food eaten throughout the day. Second, observe and record the target behavior: Keep a count of the number of times food is eaten during a 24-hour period and/or a food diary of types and amount of food eaten at each meal. Third, identify what cues the problem behavior and attempt to alter these stimuli: If overeating while watching television, avoid eating while watching television. Fourth, identify and substitute new thoughts and behaviors for old, undesirable eating habits. Fifth, identify and alter reinforcers for overeating. Recent applications of behavior modification have added the additional step of relapse prevention strategies for encouraging people to maintain their desirable behavior changes (Anderson & Creswell, 1980; Foreyt, Goodrick, Reeves, & Raynaud, 1993; Laser, 1985).

Behavioral Diagnosis
Behavioral diagnosis is based on the PRECEDE/PROCEED model of health education program planning; it involves systematic analysis and delineation of specific health-related behavioral problems that can likely affect the outcome of a health program (Gardner & Cole, 1987; Green & Kreuter, 1991; Tryon, 1976).
See **PRECEDE/PROCEED Model.**

Behavioral Epidemiology
Behavioral epidemiology, the study of individual behaviors and habits in relation to health outcomes, takes into account the role of individual behavior in causing and maintaining disease.

Example: An examination of smoking behavior and later health outcomes, such as the incidence of lung cancer (Kickbusch, 1989; Matarazzo, 1984; Owen, 1989; Wagner, 1985).

Behavioral Health

Behavioral health refers to the promotion of health by emphasizing the role behavior plays in achieving or maintaining health. Behavioral health also involves the application of behavioral and biomedical science knowledge and techniques through a variety of activities to maintain health and prevent disease (Matarazzo, Weiss, Herd, Miller, & Weiss, 1984). Behavioral health is relevant to health education and focuses on promoting health among people who are currently healthy (Rubinson & Alles, 1984; Winett, King, & Altman, 1989).

Behavioral Intention

Behavioral intention is based on Ajzen and Fishbein's (1980) Theory of Reasoned Action (recently revised to Ajzen's [1991] Theory of Planned Behavior); it is the likelihood that a person will engage in a given behavior, based on the attitudes and subjective norms held by the person (Ajzen & Fishbein, 1980; Rajecki, 1990).

To predict whether or not a person will perform a certain action you can simply ask the person. A more precise measure of likelihood may be obtained by asking the person to indicate his or her probability of carrying out the action.

Example: An individual may be asked to indicate the likelihood that she or he might abstain from sex within the next year, as follows:

I intend to abstain from sex within the next year.
Likely ___:___:___:___:___:___:___: Unlikely

Or the person may be asked to estimate the likelihood of her or his abstaining from sex within the next year in percentage points:
There is a ____% chance that I will not have sex within the next year.

See **Theory of Planned Behavior** and **Theory of Reasoned Action.**

Behavioral Medicine

Behavioral medicine is a field "concerned with the development of behavioral science knowledge and techniques relevant to the understanding of physical health and illness and the application of this knowledge and these techniques to prevention, treatment, and rehabilitation" (Rubinson & Alles, 1984, p. 247; see also Matarazzo et al., 1984).

Behavioral Objective

A behavioral objective is a statement describing precisely what the learner will be doing as a result of a learning experience. A behavioral objective is expressed in measurable terms and is also called a performance, educational, or learner objective.

Example: By the end of the program, 60% of seminar participants will commit themselves to establish a smoke-free environment at their workplace within 6 months.

Belief

A belief is a proposition or statement emotionally or intellectually accepted as true by a person or group.

Biofeedback

Biofeedback is a therapeutic method or technique used to increase awareness of a person's own physiology. On the basis of feedback from the body, one may be able to control physiological processes such as blood pressure or stress symptoms. Visual and auditory signals of changes in the biology of a person are used to make him or her aware of bodily processes of which he or she was previously unaware. As information about changes detected are fed back to the individual or patient, the person learns to control the biological system (Kaplan, 1991; Sellick & Fitzsimmons, 1989).

Biofeedback focuses on the biological systems that are beyond conscious control, but are acting in a way that impairs the individual's performance, thus contributing to stress-related diseases. In the biofeedback process, the individual first becomes aware of any faulty response, then is guided by the feedback signal to control the response, and learns to transfer this control to everyday situations.

Biofeedback is used to teach people how to relax in stress management programs and for the control of hypertension (Kaplan, Sallis, & Patterson, 1993).

Biomedical

Biomedical science is concerned with human (or animal) biology and disease, along with prevention, diagnosis, and treatment of disease.

B

Block Grant

A block grant is financial aid received by state governments from the federal government to assist cities and counties in community development, social services, education, and health. An example is the Preventive Health and Health Services Block Grant administered by the Centers for Disease Control and Prevention (CDC), which provides federal funding to all 50 states and to U.S. territories for combating chronic diseases and for health education and prevention services.

The federal government has used block grants as incentives to help the states and counties develop health services in a variety of programs, such as tuberculosis control, dental health, mental health, home health, maternal and child health, primary care, and alcohol and drug abuse prevention.

Features distinguishing block grants from other forms of federal assistance include authorizing of funds for a wide range of activities within broadly defined functional areas; giving recipient states discretion in identifying problems, designing programs, and allocating resources; and minimizing administration in fiscal reporting, planning, and other federal requirements. Block grants offer a sense of fiscal certainty to recipients.

Brainstorming

Brainstorming is a technique used in a group situation to generate as many ideas about a particular question, topic, or problem as possible in a given (usually brief) period of time. Group members are encouraged to express their thoughts spontaneously, postponing evaluation and criticism of ideas until after the brainstorming session is over.

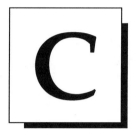

Carrier

A carrier, sometimes called *healthy carrier*, is a person or animal that harbors a specific infectious agent, but not the disease, and serves as a source of infection (Benenson, 1990).

Example: A person may carry typhoid bacillus, the infectious agent for typhoid, and although showing no symptoms of the disease or of becoming sick with typhoid, pass it to others through direct (person-to-person) or indirect (contaminated food or water; urine) contact.

Case Study

A case study is an account of a problem situation that includes sufficient information to enable meaningful discussion of contributing factors, possible preventive measures, and alternative solutions.

A case study approach to health promotion and education provides documentation of experiences to help others in the profession, particularly new entrants to the profession (Carlaw, 1982). For examples of case studies see Cleary, Kichen, and Ensor (1985).

Case Control Study

In a case control study, a group of people with a diagnosed or specified disease or problem is compared with one or more groups who do not have the same diagnosis or specified disease. Typically, case control studies are carried out retrospectively, because they often assess past exposure among cases (those with the disease) and controls (those without the disease).

C

Certification

Certification is a process by which a quasi-governmental agency or association grants recognition or licensure to a person who has met certain qualifications specified by that agency.

The National Commission for Health Education Credentialing (NCHEC) is the association responsible for granting certification to health educators. Health educators who receive certification become Certified Health Education Specialists (CHES).

See **Certified Health Education Specialist (CHES)** and **National Commission for Health Education Credentialing (NCHEC).**

Certified Health Education Specialist (CHES)

A Certified Health Education Specialist (CHES) is a person who has met all of the requirements set forth by the National Commission for Health Education Credentialing (NCHEC) and has received recognition (a certificate) as a health educator who has met the qualifications of training and experience to practice health education, and has been successful in the examination or grandfathered in by the commission. CHES after a health educator's name indicates professional competency.

See **Certification, Credentialing,** and **National Commission for Health Education Credentialing.**

Change Agent

A change agent is an individual or organization whose role is to assist other individuals or groups in identifing and dealing with issues. A change agent influences another person's decision in a direction considered desirable.

Health educators function as change agents when they work with people and encourage or influence them to make desirable changes, such as giving up smoking during pregnancy.

C

Chronic Disease

A chronic disease is a condition or health problem affecting a person for a prolonged period of time, and may result in permanent residual disability. A chronic illness may persist and become acute, ending in a crisis or death. It is a disease marked by long duration or frequent recurrence, and may require long periods of intervention or supervision.

Examples: Hypertension, diabetes mellitus, chronic respiratory problems, chronic pain, and congenital heart disease (Anderson & Bauwens, 1981).

Coalition

A coalition is a group of organizations (group of groups) in a community united to pursue a common goal. Organizations and groups join to address community issues, combining talents and resources to tackle new problems. They remain free to enter and leave at will.

A coalition may include several health agencies working together for a common good. In health education and promotion, coalitions are usually formed to deal with specific health problems in defined communities. Coalition building is essential to community-based health intervention programs and leads to increased community awareness and commitment. In addition, coalitions help to address political issues that may prevent well-planned programs from being implemented. In recent years, coalitions for smoke-free societies have been quite active, especially in California (Bracht, 1990). For additional reading on coalitions, see Green and Kreuter (1991).

Example: The Community Coalition for Substance Abuse Prevention and Treatment of Los Angeles, California, was formed to convince city and state officials that the high concentration of liquor stores in South Central Los Angeles presents a serious health hazard, and to reduce the large number of liquor licenses in that community.

Codependency

Codependency is a term used to describe individuals who are "dependent on making other people dependent on them as a means of self-validation" (Seaward, 1994, p. 97) and exhibit behaviors similar to addictive behaviors. In codependency, a person shows addiction to another person's addiction problems. Usually, the relationship between the persons is close, such as parent-child or husband-wife.

Example: Children of alcoholic parents may become codependent to their parents' addiction and problems.

Cognitive Dissonance

Cognitive dissonance is a conflict between a person's beliefs and behavior, based on Festinger's Theory of Cognitive Dissonance (Aronson, 1992; Carkenord & Bullington, 1993; Cooper, 1992; Mc Master & Lee, 1991).

Example: A person may know and believe chewing tobacco can cause mouth cancer, but may go ahead and chew anyway. The person can try to dissolve the dissonance by altering the perception of the risk or by giving up chewing.
See **Festinger's Theory of Cognitive Dissonance.**

Cognitive Domain

Cognitive domain is a category for classifying educational objectives (from Bloom's taxonomy of educational objectives for the cognitive domain) that emphasize intellectual processes, from the simplest outcomes to the most complex: knowledge, comprehension, application, analysis, synthesis, and evaluation. An objective is said to be in the cognitive domain when it requires an individual to memorize or recall facts or concepts (Bloom, 1956; Furst, 1981; Solman & Rosen, 1986).

Example: By the end of this session, the student will be able to define health education.

Cognitive Field Theory

Cognitive field theory is used mainly to explain how human behavior is learned. According to cognitive field theory, learning should not only be identified with cognition but be purposeful, explorative, and innovative.

Cognitive-Behavioral Therapy

Cognitive-behavioral therapy is a treatment approach that combines cognitive and behavioral principles to change thoughts or behavior. Cognitive-behavioral therapy may be effective in interventions for abstinence from smoking (Hall, Munoz, & Reus, 1994), panic disorder (Laberge, Gauthier, Cote, Plamonden, & Cormier, 1993), and chronic headache (James, Thorn, & Williams, 1993).

Cohort

A cohort is a group of people identified by certain characteristics or statistical factors, such as age, and followed or observed at different points over a long period of time, from exposure to outcome (Kramer, 1988; Powers & Knapp, 1990; Vogt, 1993).

A cohort is a "component of the population born during a particular time period and identified by period of birth, so that the characteristics of this group at different points in time can be identified. More generally used to describe any group of people who are followed or traced over time" (Bunton & Macdonald, 1992, p. 226).

Examples:

1. A group of coal miners ages 25-35 years being followed up for possible development of lung disease
2. Children born after the Chernobyl accident followed up for 20 years to measure radioactive iodine in the thyroid or possible radiation-induced cancers
3. A group of teenagers who began smoking in 1990 followed up over a 20-year period for possible development of lung cancer

Collaboration

Collaboration involves working together, teaming up, sharing responsibilities, or joining forces to create community intervention programs to promote health and effect behavior change or achieve goals.

Examples: School nurses may collaborate with other community service providers in an effort to meet multiple health needs of students; one nation may join forces with another nation for medical and epidemiological research (as in the case of AIDS, affecting countries worldwide); health educators may collaborate with communities for promoting primary health care and health education needs (Cowley, 1994; Handler, Schieve, Ippoliti, Gordon, & Turnock, 1994; Ritchie, 1994; Statham, 1994).

Communication

Communication is the process by which messages are transferred through a channel to a receiver and information is shared with other individuals.

See **Communication Channel.**

Communication Channel

A communication channel is the mechanism that carries information from its source to its destination, and a component of information theory. Communication channels may include interpersonal (face-to-face) communication, broadcasting (radio or television), and print (newspapers, posters, pamphlets, flyers).

See **Communication.**

Community

A community is a geographic area considered as a unit; a group of people held together by common interests or goals; or a collection of people characterized by membership (a sense of identity and belonging) or common values, language, rituals, ceremonies, needs, or history (Klein, 1968; Sarason, 1984).

A community may also be a group of people experiencing the same need, regardless of geography. A community of migrant workers scattered across the country might share the same identifiable needs.

Health educators recognize the concept of community as an integral part of community health education and health promotion (Carlaw, 1982; Carlaw & Ward, 1988). In most instances, the community can be defined as a geographical unit, such as a county, city, town, or neighborhood.

Community Development

Community development is the attempt to organize and stimulate local initiative and leadership in a community to encourage change. The emphasis in community development is on local, self-determined efforts. Community development is process oriented and emphasizes the development of skills and abilities conducive to social and health improvement (Carlaw & Ward, 1988; Rothman, 1970). Community development ideas have been used by health educators in many countries in the world to improve health, family planning, childhood nutritional status, and agriculture (Green, Kreuter, Deeds, & Partridge, 1980).

Community Empowerment

Example: By allotting garden plots to families in a village and teaching the people simple gardening techniques, a community development program on Island X was intended to help mothers grow vegetables to supplement family nutrition.

See **Community Organization.**

Community Empowerment

Community empowerment is "a social action process in which individuals and groups act to gain mastery over their lives in the context of changing their social and political environment" (Wallerstein & Bernstein, 1994, p. 142). Conceived as a health-enhancing strategy, community empowerment focuses on both individual and community change, encouraging people to listen to each other and dialogue with each other to discover new ways of looking at health problems and solutions (Israel, Checkoway, Schulz, & Zimmerman, 1994; Labonte, 1989).

Community empowerment includes the ability of people actively working together to gain understanding and control over personal, political, social, and economic forces in a community. Individuals and community organizations collectively use their skills and resources in a long-term commitment to assume more control over processes of defining problems and setting priorities in an effort to enhance health and quality of life. For additional reading on community empowerment, see the special issues on community empowerment, participatory education, and health in *Health Education Quarterly* (1994).

Community Forum

A community forum is a public meeting in which key community personnel and representatives of groups review various perspectives on, for example, health-related issues. Such forums are broad-based and encourage community involvement and participation.

Community Health

Community health is concerned with health promotion and education directed at populations rather than individuals, and involves the science and art of promoting health, preventing disease, and prolonging life through organized community effort (Lowis, 1992; Rubinson & Alles, 1984).

Community Health Education

Community health education focuses on the improvement of health and prevention of diseases within a community. Intergroup relationships, value patterns, communication resources, community organizations, policy making, strategic planning, and related methods are used to educate and mobilize community members to take actions that will enhance health and prevent disease (Rubinson & Alles, 1984).

> Community health education is the application of a variety of methods that result in the education and mobilization of community members in action for resolving health issues and problems which affect the community. These methods include, but are not limited to, group process, mass media, communication, community organization, organizational development, strategic planning, skills training, legislation, policy making, and advocacy. (1990 Joint Committee on Health Education Terminology, 1991, p. 105)

Example: The Pawtucket Health Heart Program in Rhode Island is a community-wide cardiovascular disease prevention program employing a variety of community-based interventions, targeting work sites, restaurants, schools, grocery stores, individuals, small groups, and the community at large in an effort to reduce the incidence of heart disease through screening, health education, and counseling programs directed toward risk factors such as high blood pressure, elevated cholesterol, cigarette smoking, obesity, and sedentary lifestyle (Hunt et al., 1990; Lasatar et al., 1991; Lefebvre, Lasater, Carleton, & Peterson, 1987; Schwertfeger, Elder, Cooper, Lasater, & Carleton, 1986).

Community Health Educator

A community health educator is a health professional trained in health education or public health who works in a community setting, applying a variety of methods that result in the education and mobilization of community members in actions for resolving health issues and problems that affect the community.

"A community health educator is a practitioner who is professionally prepared in the field of community/public health education who demonstrates competence in the planning, implementation, and evaluation of a broad range of health promoting or health enhancing programs for community groups" (1990 Joint Committee on Health Education Terminology, 1991, p. 105).

See **Community Health Education.**

Community Norm

Community norms are "specific rules of behavior that are agreed upon and shared within a culture to prescribe limits of acceptable behavior" (Tischler, 1993, p. 51).

Community Organization

Community organization is that process whereby community members join forces in working together to identify needs, set objectives, and take definitive action consistent with local values to develop plans for community improvement, be it in health or other matters (Rose, 1986). Health educators and advocates may play a vital role in organizing community members and groups to join forces for child and family violence reduction, or injury control.

Competitive Learning

Competitive learning is a form of learning, or learning process, in which learners compete with each other (or with themselves) to achieve certain standards of learning. It is the opposite of cooperative learning (Rumelhart & Zipser, 1985).

See **Cooperative Learning.**

Compliance

Compliance, as used in public health and health promotion, is the act of following the advice of a physician or other health care worker in a prescribed therapeutic or preventive regimen. Compliance is also referred to as *cooperation* or *adherence.*

Example: Joyce just learned that she is at high risk for coronary heart disease, and she has been given a weekly exercise regimen as a preventive measure. She complies by performing the exercises as prescribed.

Comprehensive Health Education

Comprehensive health education refers to multidimensional health programs that are usually planned and carried out by local, county, state, or federal governmental agencies with the purpose of maintaining, reinforcing, or enhancing the health, health-related skills, and health attitudes and practices of people that are conducive to their good health. It is an educational approach coordinating education, services, and environment as significant influences on individual and societal health (Bates & Winder, 1984; Rubinson & Alles, 1984; Sullivan, 1973).

Comprehensive health education is not limited to governmental agencies. Private organizations may provide comprehensive programs for a smaller community such as a workplace or school.

C

Example: A comprehensive program at the local level is the Homeless Prenatal Program (HPP) established in a San Francisco family shelter in 1989. This program provides comprehensive prenatal services to homeless pregnant women, aimed at improving their pregnancy outcomes and transforming their lives. Included in the program are good mothering techniques, prenatal care, peer support, supportive work environment, and job skills training (Ovrebo, Ryan, Jackson, & Hutchinson, 1994).

Comprehensive School Health Education

Comprehensive school health education is the planned, coordinated provision of school health services, a healthful school environment, and health instruction (education) for all learners (and staff) in a school setting in which each component complements and is integrated with the others in the total scope of the body of knowledge unique to health education (Anderson & Creswell, 1980; Brindis, 1993; Jackson, 1994; Seffrin, 1990).

Comprehensive school health education covers a variety of learning experiences appropriate to schoolchildren. It involves health education carried out in a school setting to improve health attitudes and practices, and to enhance and maintain health. Some programs also offer health education opportunities for family and community members (Cleary, 1993b; Waller & Goldman, 1993).

Comprehensive school health education aims at protecting and promoting the health and well-being of students from kindergarten through Grade 12 (Butler, 1994). Qualified teachers certified to teach in the state, together with licensed and registered nurses, provide much of the health education. Health educators may serve as health consultants, especially for the health education curriculum.

Comprehensive School Health Instruction

"Comprehensive school health instruction refers to the development, delivery and evaluation of a planned curriculum, preschool through 12, with goals, objectives, content sequence, and specific classroom lessons" (1990 Joint Committee on Health Education Terminology, 1991, p. 106). Content areas may include but are not limited to the following:

Community health
Consumer health
Environmental health
Family life and sexuality
Mental and emotional health
Injury prevention and safety
Nutrition and weight problems
Personal health
Prevention and control of disease
Substance use and abuse

Comprehensive School Health Program

A comprehensive school health education program "comprises a planned sequential prekindergarden to 12 curriculum that addresses the physical, mental, emotional, and social dimensions of health" (Allensworth & Kolbe, 1987, p. 411).

A comprehensive school health program is an organized set of policies, procedures, and activities designed to protect and promote the health and well-being of students and staff which has traditionally included health services, healthful school environment, and health education. It should also include, but not be limited to, guidance and counseling, physical education, food service, social work, psychological services, and employee health promotion. (1990 Joint Committee on Health Education Terminology, 1991, p. 105)

The term is also used in some new programs.
Comprehensive school health programs may include:

School health education
School health and nutrition services

Healthful school environment
Physical education
Psychological and counseling services
Health promotion for staff
Collaboration with parents and community

Computer-Assisted Instruction

Computer-assisted instruction involves the use of computers to teach and furnish students with information. Aimed at providing students with opportunities for putting what they learn into practice, this type of instruction can also be employed in evaluating students' achievement.

Construct Validity

Construct validity is concerned with "conformity to theoretical expectations of relationships between a previously untested measure and other variables" (Powers & Knapp, 1990, p. 25).

Consumer Behavior

Consumer behavior is "behavior that consumers display in searching for, purchasing, using, evaluating, and disposing of products, services, and ideas" (Schiffman & Kanuk, 1991, p. 651).

Consumer Health

Consumer health involves decisions that individuals make regarding the purchase and use of health products, information, and services that are available in the marketplace and can affect their health positively or negatively.

Consumer health also includes individual actions, such as the purchase of aspirins for headache or the selection of a physician, that are self-motivated and self-initiated (Cornacchia & Barrett, 1980; Schiffman & Kanuk, 1991).

Content Analysis

Content analysis is "a method for systematically and quantitatively analyzing the content of verbal and/or pictorial communication. The method is frequently used to determine prevailing social values of a society" (Schiffman & Kanuk, 1991, p. 651).

Content Outline

Content outline is a written guide that indicates the detailed process to be used for each activity listed in a lesson plan. The outline relates to the listed objectives of the lesson plan and usually incorporates the entire lesson.

Health educators often use a content outline when teaching specific health education topics to target groups at schools, colleges, universities, and community settings.

Content Validity

Content validity is "concerned with the subjective determination of validity, usually by some sort of expert judgement" (Powers & Knapp, 1990, p. 164). It refers to the degree or extent to which items or questions on a test or questionnaire are representative of the subject (Vogt, 1993).

To determine content validity, items on an instrument (questionnaire or test) should come from each content area to be measured. A review of the literature helps to establish content validity by providing comprehensive information about the topic.

Example: A health educator is the principal investigator in AIDS-related research among teenagers looking at their knowledge, attitudes, and beliefs. The questionnaire developed for this survey should include questions on each area of interest.

See **Validity.**

Contributing Factor

Contributing factors are behavioral or environmental elements that have a potential for affecting health behaviors. Contributing factors can be categorized as motivators, enablers, or reinforcers.

See **Enabling Factor** and **Reinforcing Factor.**

Cooperative Learning

Cooperative learning is characterized by learners teaching each other, sharing each other's knowledge, or working together to achieve learning goals. In public health, especially community health education, cooperative learning can be effective as peers teach peers about health. For example, teenagers can be taught the ill effects of and alternatives to tobacco smoking, and then these same teens can teach other teens by sharing what they learned. Or if health information is passed to a group regarding environmental health concepts, group members may cooperatively share this information with their peers so they can work cooperatively to improve their immediate environment. Cooperative learning is the opposite of competitive learning (Cartwright, 1993; Okebukola, 1985; Swisher, 1990).

See **Competitive Learning.**

Coping

Coping is the constantly changing cognitive and behavioral efforts that individuals make in attempts to manage specific external or internal demands that they have appraised as taxing or exceeding their resources (Antonovsky, 1980).

Most authors in the field of stress and coping recognize two primary categories: problem-focused coping and emotion-focused coping. Problem-focused coping involves taking focused action to eliminate a problem or change a situation. Emotion-focused coping includes efforts to modify impaired emotional functioning in the face of threat without trying to change the problem or situation directly.

Example: A person diagnosed with cancer (the stressor or problem) may make attempts to deal with the problem using problem-focused coping to deal directly with the cancer (seeking treatment, changing diet) and emotion-focused coping to deal with distress (attending a support group).

Cost-Benefit Analysis

Cost-benefit analysis is a measure or evaluation of the cost of an intervention relative to the benefits it yields, usually expressed as a ratio of dollars saved or gained for every dollar spent on a program.

In cost-benefit analysis, program costs and benefits are stated in monetary terms to ascertain whether the benefits exceeded the cost, even though it is difficult to place a dollar value on all program outputs (Green & Kreuter, 1991; Windsor, Baranowski, Clark, & Cutter, 1994). The potential benefits in dollars saved are divided by the cost of the intervention to provide the cost-benefit ratio.

Example: A health educator carries out a cost-benefit analysis on the cost of starting and maintaining a smoking cessation program for pregnant smokers. The cost per person enrolled will be calculated. On the benefit side, costs associated with the risk factor (smoking) include a reduction in absenteeism from work due to illness and lower medical costs to employers.

Cost-Effectiveness Analysis

Cost-effectiveness analysis is a measure or evaluation of the cost of an intervention relative to its impact, usually expressed in dollars per unit of effect. Cost-effectiveness analysis is aimed at determining the cost and effectiveness of an activity to ascertain in terms of the degree to which the objectives or outcomes are attained.

Cost-effectiveness analysis may also involve comparing programs to determine which one requires the least cost to provide the greatest level of effectiveness; the service that provides the lowest cost-per-unit benefit is the most cost-effective (Kramer, 1988).

Credentialing

Credentialing is a formal process applied to ensure that persons practicing in a profession meet minimum standards of professionalism and practice. Through credentialing, health education professionals identify and provide verification of special skills and competencies. Standards of credentialing in heath education are based on seven broad areas of responsibilities and competencies for entry-level health educators (Cleary, 1993a; Girvan, Hamburg, & Miner, 1993; Livingood et al., 1993; Mail, 1993).

See **Entry-Level Health Educator.**

The credentialing process carried out by the National Commission for Health Education Credentialing (NCHEC) includes an examination of persons who have obtained a bachelor's degree or master's degree in public health. If successful, the credentialed health educator becomes a Certified Health Education Specialist (CHES). Certification is re-newed annually through continuing education credits.

Credentialing encourages professional growth, development, and lifelong learning through continuing education opportunities.

See **Certification, Certified Health Education Specialist (CHES),** and **National Commission for Health Education Credentialing (NCHEC).**

Cross-Sectional Study

A cross-sectional study is a study of exposure and outcome in individuals or groups at a specific point in time (simultaneously). In a cross-sectional study, inferences about the differences between age groups, for example, are based on observations of people of different ages measured at the same moment. Cross-sectional designs help describe variables of interest and their distribution patterns in the population.

Example: In the Health and Nutrition Examination Survey (HANES), a sample of people was carefully selected to represent the U.S. population. The people were interviewed about their health and habits, such as the prevalence of hypertension and the average daily dietary fat intake. Comparisons are then made between groups of persons of different age, gender, race, and so forth.

C

Culture

Culture is the sum of values and traditional ideas transmitted to individuals in a community over a period of time, or patterns of behavior acquired and transmitted by human groups. Culture includes how people behave, think, and communicate their values, attitudes, beliefs, and mores (Tischler, 1993; White, 1978).

The concept of culture is important to public health and particularly health education because the cultural background, including mores, norms, and ideologies, of an individual or a community has a profound effect on their response to health education and health promotion. When designing health education programs, cultural understandings and values must be recognized in order to make the programs appropriate for the particular group.

Curriculum Guide

A curriculum guide is a written plan containing detailed information regarding health education programming. It describes the goals, philosophy, scope, and sequence of a health education program.

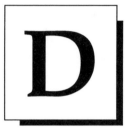

Deductive Learning

Deductive learning is a methodology in which facts and premises are assumed to be accurate and a conclusion is drawn based on these known truths. Deductive learning is the opposite of inductive learning. In the health education field, it is characterized chiefly by memorization of certain health facts presumed to lead to a change in health behavior.

Example: Adolescents taught that flossing their teeth will prevent early decay and loss of teeth acquire the facts and technique of flossing and carry out the behavior with the hope that the desired result will occur (Bedworth & Bedworth, 1992).

See **Inductive Learning.**

Delphi Technique

The Delphi technique is a method of sampling aimed at consulting and obtaining expert opinion to arrive at a consensus of planning without a face-to-face meeting. With this technique, a series of self-administered questionnaires are mailed to a number of experts, opinion leaders, or informants to establish, for example, which participants will be for a particular program or which health education program should be implemented in a community. After three or four rounds of questioning, the results are polled, tabulated, and shared. The Delphi technique, unlike the nominal group process, allows participants to present their views impersonally and confidentially without overtly influencing the opinions of others (Fish & Piercy, 1987; Reid, Peace, & Taylor, 1990; Reinke, 1988; Sarvela & McDermott, 1993).

See **Nominal Group Process.**

Dependent Variable

A dependent variable is the presumed effect or outcome being measured, and is so called because it may *depend* on manipulation of the independent variable. In public health, health educators may assess the degree to which a risk factor (obesity) affects a health outcome (heart disease), so the dependent variable depends on another variable (independent variable) and may or may not be caused by it. The dependent variable is the most important variable to an investigator.

Example: A researcher looks at the effects of participation in a weight reduction education program (independent variable) to see if there was a change or lowering of weight (dependent variable) in participants (Sarvela & McDermott, 1993). If you are studying the prevalence of heart disease among women 50 years and older, the presence of the disease is the dependent variable and age and gender are independent variables.

See **Independent Variable.**

Diagnosis

A diagnosis includes identification of causes, characteristics, signs, and symptoms of a disease or condition, and may be used as an evaluative technique to analyze health issues. In that case, it is called diagnostic evaluation. Diagnosis also refers to "information that designates or describes a health problem for the purpose of planning and evaluating interventions or establishing a prognosis" (Green & Kreuter, 1991).

Diffusion Theory

Diffusion theory provides an explanation for the diffusion of something new (an innovation) in populations, groups, individuals,

D

or social systems. Diffusion theory explains the pattern or rate of adoption of innovations by individuals or groups in a community—some persons may adopt new ideas immediately; others lag behind, but adopt at some time; and some may not adopt at all (Basch, Eveland, & Portnoy, 1986; Howze & Redman, 1992).

Diffusion theory is also known as diffusion of innovations and is a marketing principle expounded by Rogers (1983) to explain the pattern of adoption of something new. There are four components to diffusion: (a) the innovation (a program or idea that is new); (b) the channels of communication by which the program or idea is exchanged among adopters, or members of the group; (c) time; and (d) the setting or social system in which the innovation takes place (Rogers, 1983; Schiffman & Kanuk, 1991; Valente, 1993).

Many health promotion programs are thought of as innovations (something new) to specific populations, and diffusion theory helps to describe a pattern the population may follow in adopting the program (McKenzie & Jurs, 1993; Portnoy, Anderson, & Eriksen, 1989).

Example: Some people may hear of a nutrition education program to be implemented in their community and sign up to become involved without asking any questions. Others, more suspicious or less venturesome, wait until the program has started to make sure it is useful; they probably wait to receive an invitation from someone who attended the first class before signing up and attending. Still others never become involved at all.

Dose-Response Relationship

Dose-response relationship is a term used in clinical trials of drugs, but can be applicable to health promotion and education to refer to the increases in outcome measures associated with proportionate increases of resources expended. In simple terms, the more material, money, human resource initiatives, and time put into a health promotion program, the greater should be the response and resulting effects.

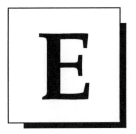

Education

Education is a complex process of experience influencing the way people perceive themselves in relation to their social and physical environments. It is a purposeful process for expediting learning.

Educational Concept

Educational concepts are summaries of the major foci of a particular lesson plan written in the learner's language. Educational concepts may also be referred to as conceptual learning.

See **Lesson Plan.**

Educational Diagnosis

An educational diagnosis is a process whereby health planners seek to assess the causes of a particular health behavior by identifying, sorting, and categorizing three classes of factors that may affect health behavior: predisposing, enabling, and reinforcing factors.

The educational diagnosis examines those behavioral and environmental conditions linked to quality of life concerns or health status to determine what causes them, and identifies factors that can be targeted for change (Gilmore, Campbell, & Becker, 1989; Sobel &

Hornbacher, 1973). In health promotion and education planning, the educational diagnosis is concerned with factors that influence behavior and living conditions of people who are at risk for identified health problems (Green & Kreuter, 1991). Educational diagnosis is Phase 4 in the PRECEDE/PROCEED model.

See **Enabling Factor, PRECEDE/PROCEED Model, Predisposing Factor,** and **Reinforcing Factor.**

Educational Goal

In general terms, educational goals are what an instructor expects to accomplish in an educational session; these goals give direction to the entire program.

Example: The participant will recognize behaviors that tend to promote health.

Educational Objective

Educational objectives are specific statements written in three domains: cognitive (acquiring knowledge and information intellectually), affective (knowledge coupled with associations such as emotions, values, and attitudes), and psychomotor (inclusion of motor skills and coordination, and development of behavioral patterns).

Example: At the conclusion of this session, the participant will be able to define high blood pressure.

Educational Tool

Educational tool is a term used interchangeably with *educational aids* and *educational materials* to refer to leaflets, videotapes, slides, bulletin boards, overhead transparencies, chalkboards, and other audiovisual support items.

Enabling Factor

Enabling factors are the skills, resources, or vehicles created by forces or systems within a society that facilitate the performance of a health action by individuals or organizations, including the availability of and access to health care, personnel, personal health skills, and outreach clinics.

Enabling factors also include barriers to action created by societal forces of systems, such as limited access to health care facilities;

inadequate resources, income, or health insurance; and restrictive laws, rules, regulations, and policies (Green & Kreuter, 1991).

Entry-Level Health Educator

In professional life, entry level is the point at which an individual becomes capable of meeting specifications for performing a role. In health education, entry level is that point at which a person has obtained the skills, knowledge, and competencies required to perform as a health educator, through a successful completion of a bachelor's, master's, or doctoral degree from an accredited college or university, with a major emphasis in health education.

There are seven areas of responsibilities and competencies for entry-level health educators, each containing a number of subcompetencies. According to A Framework for the Development of Competency-Based Curricula for Entry Level Health Educators (1985), these seven areas are:

1. Assessing individual and community needs for health education
2. Planning effective health education programs
3. Implementing health education programs
4. Evaluating effectiveness of health education programs
5. Coordinating provision of health education services
6. Acting as a resource person in health education
7. Communicating health and health education needs, concerns, and resources.

Environment

Environment encompasses the physical, social, emotional, and spiritual influences of human functioning and behavior, including animate and inanimate surroundings, and the external and internal surroundings that influence health and behavior.

Environmental Diagnosis

An environmental diagnosis includes examination of factors in the social and physical environments to determine whether or not these factors are linked to a person's behavior and identification of any impact the factors may have on behavior change. Factors outside of the individual that have a bearing on health, behavior, and quality of life include lead from paint in older homes that may cause lead

E

poisoning in children; secondhand smoke inhaled by nonsmokers, such as children in homes of smoking parents or older siblings; and gun violence and homicide (Baranowski, 1989-1990; Dever, 1976; Ross & Mico, 1980; Windsor et al., 1994). Environmental diagnosis is based on the PRECEDE/PROCEED model of health promotion planning and is often conducted along with a behavioral diagnosis (Green & Kreuter, 1991).

See **Behavioral Diagnosis, Environmental Factor,** and **PROCEED/ PRECEDE Model.**

Environmental Factor

Environmental factors include specific items or elements determined, in carrying out an environmental diagnosis, to be causally linked to health goals or quality of life problems identified in the social and epidemiological diagnoses.

Examples: Housing conditions, air, water, noise, rapid social change, crowding, and isolation.

See **Environmental Diagnosis.**

Epidemic

An epidemic is the rapid spread of a disease among individuals within a given population clearly in excess of what is normally expected. Epidemics usually affect susceptible members of a population.

Examples: The acquired immunodeficiency syndrome (AIDS) epidemic affecting all countries; the epidemic of measles among children in Dallas, Texas, in 1970 and 1971; and the plague (black death) that struck Europe during the Middle Ages (1347).

Epidemiological Diagnosis

Epidemiological diagnosis is a phase in the PRECEDE/PROCEED framework concerned with pinpointing important health problems of a target population. In health education research, epidemiological diagnosis is conducted to determine which behavioral and environmental factors contribute to the occurrence of specific targeted health problems (Green & Kreuter, 1991; Green et al., 1980).

Example: A researcher conducting an epidemiological diagnosis for a specific program gathers data such as mortality (number of people dying from the disease), morbidity (number of persons sick with the disease), incidence (new cases reported), prevalence (existing disease cases), and distribution of the health problem. Data may be gathered from statistical reports and other means available in the community. Other factors include age, sex, and ethnic group with relation to the problem being addressed.

See **Health Indicator** and **PRECEDE/PROCEED Model.**

Epidemiology

Epidemiology is the study of disease in terms of distribution, occurrence, determinants, and control in a defined human population.

Ethics

In general terms, ethics is a branch of philosophy aimed at discovering whether a conduct is good or bad or right or wrong. Ethics includes values or standards designed to shed light on the relative rightness or wrongness of actions based on moral principles, professionally endorsed and practiced.

More narrowly, ethics refers to a code or standard established by a profession to govern conduct among members. With reference to health education, the Society for Public Health Education (SOPHE) has adopted a code of ethics for health educators, who need to be aware of the ethical concerns and issues confronting them in the profession.

In 1984, a joint committee of the SOPHE and the Association for the Advancement of Health Education (AAHE) reviewed the previous code and developed a professionwide code of ethics for health education. For further information see Taub, Kreuter, Parcel, and Vitello (1987).

In 1993, SOPHE published a revised summary code of ethics, noting that "health educators take on profound responsibility in using educational processes to promote health and influence human well-being. Ethical precepts that guide these processes must reflect the right of individuals and communities to make the decisions affecting their lives." AAHE (1994) also developed health education ethics, laying out a "common set of values designed to guide health educators in resolving many of the ethical dilemmas experienced in professional life" (p. 197). These guidelines for professional conduct require from health educators a commitment to behave ethically and

E

35

to encourage and support the ethical behavior of others. (Copies of these documents can be obtained from their authors. See Part Two.)

For additional information on ethics as related to health education, see Barnes, Fors, & Becker, 1980; Greenberg & Gold, 1992; Hochbaum, 1980; Patterson & Vitello, 1993).

Etiology

Etiology is the study of the causes or origins of disease or health problems, taking into account all predisposing factors of the disease.

Example: The HIV virus that causes AIDS; a bacteria that may cause diarrhea; the tubercle bacillus that causes tuberculosis; and other factors contributing to the occurrence of disease such as poverty, environmental wastes, overcrowding, tobacco, and alcohol.

Evaluation

Broadly defined, evaluation is the comparison of an object of interest against a standard of acceptability. Evaluation can be considered as giving an account or appraisal of what has been done. This includes the level or quality of performance, suitability or appropriateness of material used, and budget constraints where applicable (Deniston & Rosenstock, 1968; Fink & Kosecoff, 1979; Windsor et al., 1994).

In the health education field, evaluation is the act of examining the worth of a program, usually measuring it against a set of predetermined objectives or a standard of acceptability. It involves the process, outcome, and impact of a program or project and demonstrates whether the program reached the desired goals and objectives. The main purpose of evaluation, with specific reference to health education programs, is to improve programs and provide feedback to professionals concerning their strengths and weaknesses, as well as to determine if objectives are being or were met, and whether people learned from the programs.

See **Formative Evaluation, Process Evaluation, Outcome Evaluation,** and **Impact Evaluation.**

Evaluation Research

Evaluation research is intended to produce evidence in support of a testable hypothesis to demonstrate convincing cause-and-effect relationships between an educational intervention and its outcome.

Evaluation research is concerned with the appraisal of the impact of an innovation on individuals or groups. It involves the application of scientific methodologies to test hypotheses concerning the impact or effectiveness of one or more interventions. One of the main objectives of evaluation research is to obtain knowledge that is generalizable in similar groups or populations in other settings (Cook & Campbell, 1979; Cook & Reichardt, 1979; Weiss, 1972; Windsor et al., 1994).

Evaluation research has been described as "an evaluation using an experimental or quasi-experimental design conducted to establish the efficacy or effectiveness—internal and/or external validity—and cost effectiveness or cost benefit of an intervention among a defined population at risk for a specific impact or outcome rate during a defined period of time" (Windsor et al., 1994, p. 15).

External Validity

External validity, also called *generalizability,* is the degree to which conclusions drawn from research or evaluation are appropriate when applied to other similar settings or populations outside the study. It is the extent to which the program or study can be applied or generalized to other populations with the expectation of producing similar effects.

Extrinsic Motivation

Extrinsic motivation is stimulating behavior by the expectation of a reward or avoidance of punishment. The concept is applicable to health promotion and education efforts to change health-related behaviors in that extrinsic motivation is often used in health education to encourage people to participate in a program.

Example: Incentives such as lotteries, drawings, raffles, or other financial rewards extrinsically motivate a person to participate in a health education program.

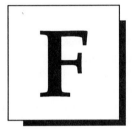

Feedback

Feedback includes verbal or nonverbal responses of a learner that the educator may interpret and use to guide learning, or a two-way communication used to evaluate the effectiveness of communication.

Festinger's Theory of Cognitive Dissonance

Festinger's (1957) theory of cognitive dissonance states that cognition or knowledge may be inharmonious to what the person does or the action a person takes. In other words, what a person does or feels may not correspond with reality, so that there is inconsistency between behavior and beliefs.

Dissonance may arise from cultural mores, specific opinions that people hold, or past experience.

Example: In one Caribbean culture, village women are fully aware that condom use can prevent unwanted pregnancy and AIDS. They are also aware of the dangers of AIDS. However, these women reject condom use because they believe that condoms are used only by men who are sick or unfaithful.

See **Cognitive Dissonance.**

Focus Group

A focus group is a type of qualitative methodology or research technique in which an experienced moderator leads a group of respondents (generally 8 to 12 persons) through an informal discussion of a selected problem or issue, allowing group members to talk freely about their thoughts, feelings, opinions, insights, attitudes, misconceptions, and beliefs about the problem. To gather information in health education research, the moderator or interviewer often uses a detailed protocol consisting of open-ended and in-depth questions (Bryant & Gulitz, 1993; Kreuger, 1989).

Focus groups are often used in needs assessment to help health educators understand why people think or act in a certain way (Graeff, Elder, & Mills-Booth, 1993). Focus groups provide an excellent opportunity for observing behavior during a needs assessment. Depending upon the topic, participants for a focus group are usually selected on the basis of certain attributes, such as students in a class, parents with disabled children, executives of major corperations, or low-income families.

See **Needs Assessment.**

Force Field Analysis

Force field analysis is a graphic examination of a problem based on Lewin's field theory, which assumes that any situation is a temporary balance between opposing forces. Driving forces that facilitate change and those that restrain change are identified and rated according to the analyzer's perception.

Formative Evaluation

Formative evaluation is evaluation undertaken in the midst of a program with the intent of using the information gained to determine program effectiveness and revise and improve the program as it is ongoing.

Formative evaluation also provides information on the kinds of outcomes that are needed and how they can be achieved. In formative evaluation, investigators look at immediate or short-term effects of a program in an effort to improve its implementation (Bedworth & Bedworth, 1992; Windsor et al., 1994).

F

Formative Research

Formative research is preliminary research conducted prior to the full planning or implementation of a research or program strategy. It may include pilot testing of a questionnaire or survey instrument to determine its acceptability. The term *formative evaluation* may be used in place of *formative research*, especially in evaluation of a program or intervention for its appropriateness and immediate impact.

Example: Rather than waiting until the end of a smoking cessation program to evaluate its effectiveness, program planners conduct formative evaluation to provide immediate feedback about the quality of the program in order to improve it while the program is ongoing. This evaluation would include information from a variety of sources, such as program participants and program providers both before and during program implementation.

See **Pilot Testing.**

F

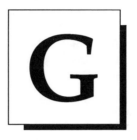

Gannt Chart

A Gannt chart is a timetable that shows each activity in a program plan on a horizontal line that extends from the beginning to the finish date. A program manager can use this chart at any given time to see the activities that are about to begin, those that are taking place, and those due to be completed (see chart below).

ACTIVITIES	MAY-JUN	SEPT-AUG	SEP-OCT	NOV-DEC
Preliminary planning	X			
Data collection	X			
Data analysis		X		
Program planning			X	
Material production			X	
Recruitment/training			X	
Implement program				X
Program evaluation				X

Gatekeeper

A gatekeeper is a person with whom one must work to reach a target audience or accomplish a task. Gatekeepers act as intermediaries between those promoting health and those to whom the health message is being directed; they include community leaders, clergy, and parents (Dorken, 1989; Emlet & Hall, 1991; Wallston, Hoover-Dempsey, Brissie, & Rozee-Koker, 1989).

Examples: Working with a schoolteacher or principal before implementing a program for schoolchildren; in some cultures, working with husbands prior to implementing family planning education for wives in a community.

Generational Epidemic

Generational epidemics are health and other problems perpetuated from parents to offspring.

Examples: Many alcoholics are children of alcoholics; a number of child abusers are victims of child abuse.

G

Goal

A goal is a statement of broad intent that provides direction in making program decisions—a long-range target toward which behavior change is directed. Goals describe desired levels of resources and expected outcomes, or what should happen as a result of, for example, health education programs. Goals are global expectations formulated to include all components of a program.

Examples:

1. The goal of this program is to enhance the lives of children by teaching them to make food choices that may lower their risk of heart disease.
2. The goal of this program is to develop a child bicycle helmet intervention aimed at reducing head injuries in children.

Group Dynamics

Group dynamics is the process of interaction between a person and other members of a group; group interaction is concerned with the effect of a group upon an individual's readiness to change or maintain, for example, certain health standards or norms.

Group Process

Group process applies educational and communication principles in group situations. Group process can facilitate problem solving and decision making through creative thinking to increase credibility and acceptance of recommended health practices.

G

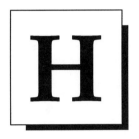

Health

Health, as defined by the World Health Organization (WHO), is a "complete state of physical, mental, and social well-being, and not merely the absence of disease or infirmity."

Health may be defined as the quality of a person's physical, psychological, and sociological functioning that enables him or her to deal with a variety of personal and social situations (Bedworth & Bedworth, 1992).

"Health is the capacity to cope with or adapt to disruptions among the organic, social, and personal components of the individual's health system" (Bates & Winder, 1984, p. 36).

Health Advising

"Health advising is a process of informing and assisting individuals or groups in making decisions and solving problems related to health" (1990 Joint Committee on Health Education Terminology, 1991, p. 105).

Health Advocacy

Health advocacy is the employment of specific approaches, guidelines, resources, and strategies to bring about social or organizational change on behalf of a particular interest group or population, and to influence policy choices, public or private (Carey, Chapman, & Gaffney, 1994; Howze & Redman, 1992; Lupton, 1994; Nyswander, 1967).

Advocacy is one of the common strategies used in the organization of community members and decision makers to address barriers that impede successful health education intervention.

Example: A group of health professionals takes a position on the issue of cigarette advertising on billboards that target minority communities and initiates actions to influence the public and policymakers to design laws prohibiting such billboards in those communities.

Labonte (1994) identifies three facets in advocacy in health professional practice. Professionals can offer health-related knowledge and analytical skills to already established community advocacy groups; health institutions can play a role in legitimizing advocacy concerns of community groups by helping to create appropriate policy documents and defining the importance of social life through the services they offer; and finally, health professionals can take a position on public health policy issues at the local, state, or national government levels, including current social welfare reforms, community housing needs, and pertinent environmental standards.

Health Agency

A health agency is a government or private organization established for the protection and improvement of people's health, such as the World Health Organization (WHO), the National Institute of Health (NIH), a Ministry of Health, county departments of health, the Centers for Disease Control and Prevention (CDC), the National Kidney Foundation, and the Epilepsy Foundation of America.

Health agencies maintain vital health records; monitor disease; and provide direct services and health education to clients through workshops, seminars, and printed materials.

H

Health Behavior

Health behavior is behavior directed at reducing disease risks and early death, and includes personal attributes such as beliefs, expectations, values, perceptions, prevention, behavior patterns, actions, and habits that relate to health maintenance, restoration, and improvement. Living conditions, eating habits, and exercise habits, and other activities undertaken to prevent disease are also relevant (Bedworth & Bedworth, 1992; Glanz, Lewis, & Rimer, 1990; Green & Kreuter, 1991).

Health Belief Model (HBM)

The Health Belief Model, first developed by a group of psychologists to help explain why people did or did not use health services (Becker, 1974; Rosenstock, 1974, 1991), is a theoretical model according to which behavior is a function of knowledge, beliefs, and attitudes.

The Health Belief Model describes and predicts health behavior in terms of beliefs and perceptions about illness, cost of care, and benefits that may accrue. This model is frequently used by health educators in health behavior applications to predict, describe, and explain health-related behavior based on a person's perceptions and belief patterns. The model is based on the assumption that a person must believe that he or she will develop a health problem in order to take action. The main influences on behavior are perceived susceptibility to a disease, perceived severity of a disease, perceived costs and benefits of taking preventive action, perceived barriers to taking action, and cues to action (advice from peers, mass media campaigns, illness of family member, or newspaper article relating to the problem). There must be sufficient concern for health on the individual's part to make health issues relevant.

Health Benefit

A health benefit is a valued improvement or outcome in quality of life that can be attributed to the process of health care.

Example: A person with a heart problem attends a live-in cardiovascular health promotion program involving nutrition, exercise, and other health-related practices and receives the benefit of extending life expectancy without a major heart attack for several years.

Health Care Delivery System

A health care delivery system is an organized system of services, equipment, personnel, and facilities through which individuals, families, or communities receive health care, including diagnosis; treatment and preventive measures; and patient education for the purpose of promoting, maintaining, and restoring health.

The Loma Linda Centers for Health Promotion and the Kaiser Permanente health care system include health promotion, education, and preventive services. In these systems, participants are diagnosed; treated; and placed in preventive care and health maintenance programs involving dietary changes, weight loss, smoking cessation, periodic screening, exercise, immunization, and other practices that may help to restore or maintain health.

Health Care Provider

Health care providers include nurses, physicians, dentists, podiatrists, physical therapists, occupational therapists, psychologists, paramedics, optometrists, health educators, practical nurses, nurse practitioners, physician assistants, village health workers, dental hygienists, speech therapists, dietitians, nutritionists, certain health care corporations, and others who take care of persons needing some form of medical or psychological help.

Health Communication

As defined by CDC, "health communication is the crafting and delivery of messages and strategies, based on consumer research, to promote the health of individuals and communities" (Roper, 1993, p. 179).

Aimed at influencing individual behavior and reducing health risks, health communication involves a series of successive stages such as examining background information to see what exists in the community, setting communication objectives, analyzing and segmenting target audiences, developing and pretesting messages to be communicated to consumers, selecting channels of communication (*see* **Communication Channel**), developing a plan for communication activities, implementing the communication strategy, evaluating the effectiveness of the activities, and providing feedback for improvement and more effective planning.

H

Health Consultant

A health consultant is a technical expert in the field of health education, health promotion, health administration, or health services who has influence in planning and advising on health matters, but no direct power to make changes.

Health consultants may be called in by private health organizations, schools, colleges, government health departments, and ministries of health in foreign countries to work with committees and health professionals advising on health matters and possible programs or projects to be planned and implemented.

Health Counseling

Health counseling consists of procedures by which health educators, nurses, physicians, other health professionals, agencies, and organizations interpret a health problem to learners or others as a means of helping them find a solution.

Health counseling may be carried out on an individual or group basis depending on the situation (Bedworth & Bedworth, 1992).

Example: A person who has been diagnosed with hypertension and has a family history of the disease is referred to a health educator or nurse, who explains and interprets what hypertension is all about, the importance of taking action to prevent early disability, the types of foods to include in or delete from the diet, the benefits of exercise, and sources for additional help.

A survey on the effectiveness of clinical interventions to prevent disease concluded that overall, counseling may be more valuable than conventional clinical activities in preventing disease. Counseling by health professionals is effective in helping people change dietary, smoking, and other behaviors that negatively affect health (U.S. Preventive Services Task Force, 1989).

Health Education

Health education is an educational process concerned with providing a combination of approaches to lifestyle change that can assist individuals, families, and communities in making informed decisions on matters that affect restoration, achievement, and maintenance of health.

H

Health education is also a deliberately structured discipline or profession that provides learning opportunities about health through interactions between educators and learners using a variety of learning experiences. This process of learning can enable people to voluntarily change conditions or modify behavior (*see* **Behavior Modification**) for health enhancement (*see* **Health Enhancement**).

Health education is much more than factual information. It includes all those experiences that affect the way people think and feel about their health, and it motivates them to put information into practice (Bates & Winder, 1984; Bedworth & Bedworth, 1992; Greenberg, 1992; Rubinson & Alles, 1984).

Health Education Administrator

A health education administrator is a person trained in health, health education, education, and administration who combines these skills in organizing, administering, supervising, and evaluating health education programs.

Health education administrators are concerned with providing direction and leadership to a health agency (voluntary or governmental) or a school, and seeing that program goals are achieved. They also organize health education programs on the district, community, and state level.

Health education administrators should have training and experience in health administration and a working knowledge of health education and its relationship to the health care system, and they must be able to use effective communication. For role delineation, functions, and responsibilities, see Bedworth and Bedworth (1992, chap. 10).

H

Examples:

1. School Health Education Administrator (functions at a city, county, and state level).
2. Health Education Administrator (may function in health departments, hospitals, or HMOs in charge of the health education department).

Health Education Coordinator

"A health education coordinator is a professional health educator who is responsible for the management and coordination of all health education policies, activities, and resources within a particular setting or circumstance" (1990 Joint Committee on Health Education Terminology, 1991, p. 104).

Health Education Curriculum Guide

A health education curriculum guide is a tool developed or designed in broad terms to include such items as family living, drugs, growth and development, nutrition, safety, environment, community health, and mental health. This guide is used to plan courses to encourage positive health attitudes and behavior in students, helping them to better understand health problems and issues, and to integrate concepts associated with physical, mental, social, spiritual, and emotional well-being. A health education curriculum guide should be flexible to allow for adaptation in individual school districts.

Health Education Diagnosis

Health education diagnosis is the identification and delineation of factors that predispose, enable, or reinforce a specific health behavior in a person or population. It is also referred to as *educational diagnosis* in the PRECEDE/PROCEED model.

See **Educational Diagnosis** and **PRECEDE/PROCEED Model.**

Health Education Field

The health education field is the multidisciplinary practice concerned with planning, implementing, and evaluating health education programs that are intended to empower individuals, families, communities, and community organizations to achieve, protect, and sustain health.

Health Education Policy

A health education policy is a plan of action focused on fostering the development of health promotion programs, including training and utilization of health education personnel.

With the increased use of health education in treatment and illness prevention, as well as the focus on personal health behaviors and practice, health educators are involved in policy making pertinent to specific programs or projects (Davis, 1985; Mico, 1978; Simonds, 1978).

Health Education Practice

Health education practice is the application of knowledge and skills based on educational theories to promote health and lifestyle changes in a target population.

Examples: Conducting a weight loss program, an antidrug campaign, or teaching cancer prevention education to high-risk groups. *See* **Health Education.**

Health Education Process

Health education process is the continuum or series of learning experiences that enables people to make decisions, modify behaviors, and change social and environmental conditions to be more conducive to health enhancement.

Example: Providing opportunities for pregnant teenagers to receive prenatal education and promoting breast-feeding.

Health Education Program

A health education program is a planned combination of activities based on needs assessment, broad principles of education, and evaluation targeted at a population. A health education program usually involves the setting of goals and objectives and is geared to a specific population.

Example: The Hale County Cancer Communication Program, established in the 1970s by the Alabama Department of Public Health, with the intent of reaching rural poor minority (Black) women more than 35 years of age who had never had a Pap smear. Among the intervention techniques was the establishment of clinics for screening and the training of female lay leaders to conduct programs for women's groups with the intent of increasing the number of women visiting the screening clinics and participating in the program (Windsor et al., 1994).

Health Education Standards

Health education standards specify what students in the health education profession should know and be able to do. Knowledge and skills essential to the development of health literacy include the ways of communicating, reasoning, and investigating that characterize

H

health education. Health education standards are *not* merely facts. Rather, they identify the knowledge and skills students should master in order to attain a high level of competency in health education. Skills may include problem solving, decision making, critical thinking, health literacy, mathematical skills, and the ability to collaborate and apply knowledge from multiple content areas in a work setting. The ultimate goal of health education standards is improved education for students and improved health in the United States. It is anticipated that standards in health education will help achieve the health promotion goals in *Healthy People 2000: National Health Promotion and Disease Prevention Objectives* (Public Health Service, 1990). (A copy of the booklet with the Health Education Standards can be purchased from the Association for the Advancement of Health Education or the American Cancer Society.)

Health Education Tool

A health education tool is any material or teaching aid, such as films, videos, slides, overhead transparencies, or pamphlets, designed to improve the learning process. Tools include spot advertisements on television and radio.

See **Educational Tool.**

Health Educator

A health educator is an individual who specializes in health education through academic preparation and assists other individuals in making informed decisions in matters affecting their health.

"A health educator is a highly trained individual who attempts to improve the health of people through use of the educational process" (Bedworth & Bedworth, 1992, p. 447). A health educator may have specialized interests such as community health, school health, patient education, or cooperative or work site health education.

"A health educator is a practitioner who is professionally prepared in the field of health education, who demonstrates competence in both theory and practice, and who accepts responsibility to advance the aims of the health education profession" (1990 Joint Committee on Health Education Terminology, 1991, p. 103).

A health educator may function in a variety of settings, such as community health agencies, public health agencies, work sites, schools, colleges, universities, hospitals, clinics, voluntary health organizations, health maintenance organizations, professional organizations, and other organizations and agencies with a health education emphasis or program. Persons from diverse backgrounds, such as nurses, physicians, social workers, and educators, may also become health educators and function within the field or include health promotion and education as a component of their work.

Health Enhancement

Health enhancement is a dimension of health promotion pertaining to the aim of reaching higher levels of wellness beyond the mere absence of disease and infirmity. Health enhancement begins with people who are basically healthy, but it is not limited to the well population. Persons with chronic diseases such as cardiovascular problems may be provided with exercise facilities and encouraged to exercise regularly in order to improve their level of wellness (Chenoweth, 1991).

Health Equity

Health equity is the concept that ideally everyone should have a fair opportunity to achieve full health potential and that equal opportunities for health should be created to lower health differentials among individuals or groups. Unfortunately, this concept of fair and equal opportunity in health care for everyone has not been achieved in the United States, and does not presently seem likely given the problems of access to health care, available resources, and ethnic concerns.

See **Access to Health Care.**

Health Facility

A health facility is a setting such as a building, health education center, health clinic, hospital, nursing home, sports medicine clinic, weight loss clinic, or other similar places where health care is provided and health resources are possible.

Health Fair

A health fair is a community health promotion program set up in a mall, hall, or other place frequented by consumers. Health fairs are also conducted at work sites for employees and their families. Booths are used to demonstrate information on cholesterol, hypertension, diabetes, dental screening and care, weight control, and nutrition in relation to specific conditions and diseases. Videos, films, audiovisual

H

displays, exhibits, pamphlets, handouts, and other health-related material can help raise the level of consciousness about health issues among members of the community. Other areas of health interest may be included as appropriate to the specific community.

Participants in a health fair may be drawn from community groups including the county health department; churches; schools; work sites; hospitals; fire and police departments; medical and dental auxiliaries; health agencies; and associations such as the American Cancer Society, the American Heart Association, and the American Lung Association (Breckon, Harvey, & Lancaster, 1989, 1994; Chenoweth, 1991).

Health Indicator

A health indicator is a marker of a health problem, such as mortality (e.g., number of female deaths from all causes per 100,000 population), morbidity (e.g., number of people with a chronic disease such as diabetes, or number of children under 10 years of age with anemia), or disability (e.g., number of persons incapacitated or disadvantaged sufficiently to warrant special care), that gives clues to life expectancy.

Health indicators are essential to health agencies, health departments, and countries attempting to control disease, and to health educators and health care workers in planning health education and public health activities (Lilienfeld & Lilienfeld, 1980).

See **Morbidity** and **Mortality.**

H

Health Information

"Health information is the content of communications based on data derived from systematic and scientific methods as they relate to health issues, policies, programs, services, and other aspects of individual and public health, which can be used for informing various populations and in planning health education activities" (1990 Joint Committee on Health Education Terminology, 1991, p. 104).

Health Information System

A health information system is a data collection scheme to provide information about the impact of a health education program and the effect it is having on its target group or community. Data collected are saved for retrieval as needed for research, teaching, statistical information, and program evaluation.

Example: A county health agency can retrieve data from a health information system to help with assessing the community needs and identifying specific effects of past projects.

Health Literacy

"Health literacy is the capacity of an individual to obtain, interpret, and understand basic health information and services and the competence to use such information and services in ways which are health enhancing" (1990 Joint Committee on Health Education Terminology, 1991, p. 104).

Health Maintenance Organization (HMO)

A health maintenance organization (HMO) is an organized prepaid health care delivery system, public or private, set up to provide health care maintenance and treatment services in a geographic area. The idea dates back to the late 1940s with the Kaiser Foundation health plan. Payment to an HMO is usually through a reimbursement plan of predetermined periodic prepayments made by or on behalf of participating individuals (Kress & Singer, 1975).

HMOs were created with the intention of setting up a new system of health care delivery at a time when the cost of health care exceeded the means of many Americans, as remains the case today. HMOs focus on reducing health care cost and incorporating health education and promotion as an integral part of the medical system.

Most HMOs contract with independent physicians or employ physicians of various specialties. The physicians may be paid a salary or a flat fee for each patient per month. Typically, an employer pays a fixed fee in return for all necessary health care for employees, who may or may not be required to make a copayment. To control cost, reimbursements may be by patients' diagnoses rather than their length of stay in the facility. Thus a hospital on the HMO system would be paid a fixed fee for each cancer patient or heart attack patient, regardless of how long the patient was hospitalized. Because of this patients may be moved out of hospitals more promptly to increase the volume of patients using the service. The Kaiser Permanente hospitals and Group Health Cooperative are two of the major players in this system of prepaid group health (Bedworth & Bedworth, 1992; Kaplan et al., 1993; Kotler, 1975; Langwell, 1990; Mielke, 1994).

H

Health Outcome

Health outcome is a specified change, positive or negative, in an individual, patient, or population that results from health promotion or health care. It includes results from the impact of a program on participants, and an examination of whether new behavior is associated with improved health or whether changes in behavior led to health status outcomes.

Example: Health educators conduct a needs assessment to determine what programs ought to be offered in a community and as a result select a prenatal education program for teenage mothers. In this program, health outcomes may include lower medical cost, fewer babies with low birth weight, fewer pregnancy complications, fewer Caesarean sections, and shorter hospital stays.

For additional reading on health outcomes, see Windsor et al. (1994, pp. 66-67).

See **Impact Evaluation.**

Health Outcome Evaluation

An outcome evaluation is "designed to assess intervention efficacy or effectiveness in producing long-term changes (e.g., 1-10 years) in the incidence or prevalence of morbidity rates, mortality rates, or other health status indicators for a clinically diagnosed medical condition among a defined population at risk" (Windsor et al., 1994, p. 14).

H

Health Policy

A health policy is a health-directed plan of action designed to influence the delivery of health care services, and includes a written document to help regulate health care, health services, and health programs.

The health policy process involves input from federal, state, and local governments, legislative and executive bodies, advocacy groups, corporations, independent agencies, insurers, health care providers, the media, and educational institutions.

Health policy is being employed in decision making on several health promotion and education issues, and many health behavior problems have serious implications for policy. Health policy formation and implementation interrelate with the behaviors, attitudes, and knowledge of the public in matters affecting health.

Example: The case of Kimberly Bergalis and four other patients who apparently became infected with the human immunodeficiency virus (HIV) in a dentist's office during a course of treatment resulted in proposals for risk prevention policy decisions such as the use of masks, gloves, and other protective gear, as well as more stringent sterilization regarding HIV-infected health care professionals (Glantz, Mariner, & Annas, 1992; Steckler & Dawson, 1982).

Health educators need an adequate understanding of the development of policy, and should participate in policymaking whenever opportunities arise. Health educators are valuable resource persons in the role of health policy formation.

Health Problem

A health problem includes any condition of being unsound in body, mind, or spirit that adversely affects the quality of life.

Health Promotion

Health promotion is the use of a combination of health education and specific interventions, such as antismoking campaigns, breast health month, and diabetes awareness, at the primary level of prevention designed to facilitate behavioral and environmental changes conducive to health enhancement.

Health promotion aims at helping people change their lifestyle through public participation in a combination of efforts to enhance awareness and create environments that support positive health practices that may result in reducing health risks in a population (Bunton & Macdonald, 1992; Green & Kreuter, 1991; Seymour, 1984; Tannahill, 1985).

Health promotion involves three levels of attempts to improve and maintain health:

1. Disease prevention
2. Health enhancement
3. Medical care

Health promotion can occur in various settings, such as the community as a whole, hospitals, clinics, churches, organizations such as the Young Men's Christian Association (YMCA) and the Young Women's Christian Association (YWCA), community wellness centers, schools, and work sites.

H

57

Health Protection

Tasks include needs assessment, problem identification, development of appropriate goals and objectives, creation of interventions, implementation of interventions, and the evaluation of outcomes or results. Benefits of health promotion information may include change in attitudes, increased awareness and knowledge, lowered risk for certain health problems, better health status, and improved quality of life.

Examples: Dental Health Awareness Week, Alcohol Awareness Month, Employee Fitness Month, Cancer Prevention Week, tobacco cessation programs, and drug awareness seminars.

Professionals who engage in health promotion may include health educators, nurses, physicians, physical therapists, dentists, dental hygienists, social workers, teachers, and nutritionists.

Health Protection

Health protection involves strategies that focus on environmental rather than on behavioral determinants of health. Emphasis is therefore given to providing a wholesome environment with the hope of protecting the health of individuals and communities. Specific areas targeted in today's society are the following:

1. Environmental hazards such as toxic waste sites, industrial chemicals, and exposure to lead, air pollutants, and radon.
2. Food and drug safety, with special interest in pesticide residues and microbial contamination.
3. Occupational health and safety, such as wearing protective clothing, goggles, and gloves when working with dangerous chemicals and monitoring workplaces for emerging hazards.
4. Unintentional injuries including motor vehicle collisions, falls, drownings, poisonings, and residential fires. Protection from unintentional injuries focuses on stopping drunk driving and promoting the use of protective helmets, seat belts, and other safety mechanisms.

Health Risk Appraisal

Health risk appraisals are computer software programs specially prepared and widely used to compute and determine health risks of individuals and needs of targeted populations. They are instruments requiring people to respond to a number of questions about their

H

health behavior and health history, and may include clinical screening such as height, weight, blood pressure, and cholesterol measurements. The information is usually entered into a computer program designed to provide individual and group results. Results from appraisals may be used to suggest risk-reduction activities—reducing weight to normal range, stopping smoking, decreasing use of high fat and high cholesterol foods, and increased exercise.

Health appraisals can be used with students (college and university), employees at work sites in business and industry, hospitals, and clubs to help prioritize needs and plan appropriate programs.

Health Status

Health status is the measured state of an individual's health or that of a population. An individual's health can be measured by weight, height, blood pressure, heart rate, family health history, and lifestyle practices regarding smoking or exercise. In measuring the health status of a population, one may want to look beyond these measurements to data and trends about disease, including incidence and prevalence rates, mortality and morbidity data, and environmental factors that may enhance or adversely affect health (Bates & Winder, 1984).

Health-Directed Behavior

Health-directed behavior, also referred to as *health behavior*, involves actions deliberately aimed at protecting or improving one's health.

Examples: Adopting a low-fat or low-salt diet or a diet containing less meat; the decision to assign a sober driver if the designated driver was drinking alcohol; wearing bicycle helmets and seat belts.

See **Health Behavior.**

Healthful School Environment

A healthful school environment includes safe and clean school buildings, parking lots, swimming pools, playgrounds, rest rooms, locker rooms, and science laboratories. Also important are clean food preparation and serving areas, adequate classroom lighting, ventilation, and noise control, as well as protection against radiation, asbestos, and lead. In addition, safety requires adequate disposal of toxic and other waste material, smoke-free classrooms, drug-free school

H

grounds, and avoidance of crime and violence. The health environment forms the basis for other health services development.

Healthy Lifestyle

"Healthy lifestyle is a set of self-enhancing behaviors, shaped by internally consistent values, attitudes, beliefs, and external social and cultural forces" (1990 Joint Committee on Health Education Terminology, 1991, p. 102).

Healthy People 2000

Healthy People 2000 (Public Health Service, 1990) is an influential U.S. government report that set forth national health promotion and disease prevention goals for the year 2000. The report lays out a framework and directs national attention to realistic opportunities to achieve a healthier nation by the year 2000. The report states clearly that achievement depends on acceptance of shared responsibilities among governments at every level, the media, health professionals, communities, families, and individuals. It is a national consensus of health improvements expected to be achieved through concerted public and private effort, and provides a platform for action.

Healthy People 2000 grew out of a health strategy initiated in 1979 with the publication of *Healthy People: The Surgeon General's Report on Health Promotion and Disease Prevention* (U.S. Surgeon General, 1979). This report showed the dramatic gains that had been achieved in the United States since the turn of the century and what was required for continued improvement. National public health goals were set according to age group with targeted declines in mortality to be reached by 1990.

Three broad goals were formulated in *Healthy People 2000:*

1. Increase the life span of healthy life for Americans. The concept is that long life without health is insufficient.
2. Reduce health disparities among Americans. Special attention was placed on reducing and eventually eliminating disparities in death, disease, and disability rates among population groups, with specific reference to those who have been disadvantaged economically, educationally, and politically.
3. Achieve access to preventive services for all Americans. Access to preventive services includes an increase in the number of persons

who have a source of primary health care and adequate insurance for primary as well as preventive care.

To support these major goals, *Healthy People 2000* lists 300 measurable objectives organized in 22 priority areas. Of these 22 priority areas, 21 fall into three broad sections—health promotion, health protection, and preventive services (see entries)—and one cuts across all categories and addresses surveillance and data systems.

Examples of Healthy People 2000 *objectives:*

1. Increase to at least 75% the proportion of work sites with a formal smoking policy that prohibits or severely restricts smoking at the workplace. (Baseline: 27% of work sites with 50 or more employees in 1985; 54% of medium- and large-sized companies in 1987.)
2. Reduce deaths caused by alcohol-related motor vehicle collisions to not more than 8.5 per 100,000 people. (Age-adjusted baseline: 9.8 per 100,000 in 1987.)

For additional reading and a complete list of the *Healthy People 2000* National Health Promotion and Disease Prevention Objectives, see *Healthy People 2000,* which can be obtained from libraries or the Government Printing Office.

H

Hierarchy of Learning
Hierarchy of learning projects three levels of progressive learning:

1. The acquisition of health facts, which may include knowledge about certain health issues or the cause and prevention of certain health problems
2. The development of health attitudes, or feelings about a health problem
3. The development of values that may lead to behavior change

Health educators are well aware that the acquisition of knowledge (health facts) does not necessarily ensure proper health behavior. Health educators must concern themselves with learning situations such as attitudes, beliefs, and values in addition to knowledge (Bedworth & Bedworth, 1992).

Hierarchy of Needs

Hierarchy of needs is a concept developed in the 1950s by Abraham Maslow, who arranged needs in an order of importance from the most basic biological needs to psychological needs concerned with self-actualization, with the assumption that needs lower down in the hierarchy must be met before the motivation to meet higher needs manifests (Lester, 1990; Lester, Hvezda, Sullivan, & Plourde, 1983; Strong & Fiebert, 1987; Williams & Page, 1989).

There are five basic needs, ranging from lowest to highest (hierarchically):

1. Physiological—the need for such basics as food, water, and oxygen
2. Safety—the need for protection
3. Love—the need for a feeling of belonging
4. Esteem—the need to feel appreciated
5. Self-actualization—the need to achieve one's full potential in terms of growth, development, and functioning

The hierarchy of needs concept is important to health educators, especially those involved in counseling, who must often address issues of self-esteem, safety, and self-actualization (Bedworth & Bedworth, 1992).

H

Host

A host is a person or animal (including birds and arthropods) who harbors a disease or condition. A squirrel may carry rabies, or cattle may act as host for certain tick-borne disease. A host may be identified in different ways: A host in which the parasite attains maturity or passes its sexual stage is considered primary; a host in which a parasite is in a larval or asexual state is referred to as intermediate or secondary; and a host in which the organism remains alive but does not undergo development is a transport host.

See **Carrier.**

Hypothesis

A hypothesis is a supposition or prediction that an investigator sets out to prove. It is a tentative statement postulating that a relationship exists between two or more variables or characteristics (Creswell,

1994; Kramer, 1988), such as smoking (exposure to tar and other chemicals in cigarettes) and lung cancer (a disease).

A hypothesis may be expressed in the "null" form (e.g., there is no relationship between hormone therapy and breast cancer in menopausal women) or in the "alternative" form (e.g., the more that menopausal women use hormone therapy, the more likely it is that they will develop breast cancer).

In scientific research and evaluation, a hypothesis is a prediction of the results of an experiment or study; a tentative proposition to be confirmed or rejected by research (Powers & Knapp, 1990).

Example: On the issue of AIDS and teenagers, a hypothesis statement could be, "There is no relationship between teenagers' perception of risk of AIDS and their intended sexual behavior." This hypothesis could be tested by collecting data or facts from teenagers regarding their perception of risk for getting AIDS and their behavior intention. These facts will lead to the acceptance or rejection of the hypothesis through determining whether or not a relationship between the two variables exists (Creswell, 1994; Kramer, 1988; Powers & Knapp, 1990).

H

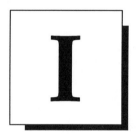

Illness Behavior

Illness behavior, as distinguished from health behavior, refers to activities undertaken by persons who feel ill to discover what is wrong and what can be done about it. Illness refers to what the person feels is wrong and not what a doctor says or discovers is amiss (Alonzo, 1984; Frankel & Nuttall, 1984; Lipkin, 1980; Wooley, Blackwell, & Winget, 1978).

Example: A person may feel ill and visit a health screening and consultation program and take height and weight measurements, blood pressure tests, urine tests, and possibly an electrocardiogram (ECG or EKG) to discover why she or he feels ill and to help plan a course of action.

See **Health Behavior.**

Impact Evaluation

Impact evaluation is an assessment of the immediate or midterm effects that a program or some aspect of a program had on the target behaviors (Windsor et al., 1994; Windsor, Kronenfeld, Ory, & Kilgo, 1980). Impact evaluation is designed to determine whether a project's objectives have been achieved and whether changes that were observed in the population can be attributed to efforts generated by the program.

Example: A number of people began using condoms after the first session of a promotion program. Impact evaluation looks at the program objectives for immediate changes in predisposing, enabling, reinforcing, behavioral, and environmental factors (Green & Kreuter, 1991; Windsor et al., 1994).

See **Enabling Factor, Environmental Factor, Outcome Evaluation, Predisposing Factor, Program Evaluation,** and **Reinforcing Factor.**

Incentive

An incentive is a commodity or condition capable of stimulating action to satisfy a drive or achieve goals. An incentive is often used as an extrinsic motivational device that may take the form of reward or punishment.

An incentive is something that an individual looks forward to upon completion of a task—a reward. An incentive that is perceived as positive is usually more desirable and effective than one perceived as negative.

Incentives are important in motivating behavior, and in this sense, health behavior, but only to the extent that they relate to previous similar behavior. If the incentive used is unfamiliar to the individual it may be meaningless.

Example: A person may be offered free exercise equipment as a reward for completing a 6-week intensive course of exercise and physical fitness, or a trip to the Bahamas for losing 20 pounds.

I

Incidence

Incidence is a measure of new cases of a disease, or the frequency of occurrence of a disease based on new cases in a population within a certain time period. It is the number of instances of persons falling ill during a given time in a specified population.

Incidence is often used to indicate incidence rate—the rate at which new events (cases) occur in a population or an estimate of the probability (risk) of people developing a disease during a specified period of time. In public health, incidence is used as a measurement of morbidity, or to express morbidity, and is calculated by dividing the number of new cases over a specified period of time by the population at risk and presented as follows:

$$\text{Incidence rate per 1,000} = \frac{\text{Number of new cases of a disease occurring in the population during a specified period of time}}{\text{Number of persons exposed to risk of developing the disease during that period of time}} \times 1,000$$

Health educators and public health workers need to be aware of the incidence or occurrence of disease in a population to plan appropriate and effective interventions.

Independent Variable

An independent variable is the presumed cause of a phenomenon that can be used to predict the value of another variable. An independent variable causes a change in something. In an experiment the researcher manipulates the independent variable in order to observe its effects on the dependent variable. The independent variable is also referred to as the predictor variable in epidemiological research (Friedman, 1980; Powers & Knapp, 1990; Vogt, 1993).

Example: To better understand the relationship between obesity and heart disease, weight reduction must also be considered. Participation in a weight reduction program or weight loss (independent variable), may reduce heart disease (dependent variable) in specific individuals.

See **Dependent Variable.**

Inductive Learning

Inductive learning is a methodology of learning from examples. The method begins with a question such as, "What factors predispose a person to developing hypertension?" or a hypothesis statement such as, "There is no relationship between cigarette smoking and hypertension." This is followed by the accumulation of empirical evidence or discoveries, from which conclusions are drawn (Bunting, 1981; Holyoak, Koh, & Nisbett, 1989; Lee, 1982).

In relation to health education, inductive learning methodology begins with a health problem or issue, followed by an accumulation of empirical evidence, from which conclusions, facts, and answers are drawn or learned. This method of learning is the opposite of deductive learning.

See **Deductive Learning.**

Information Theory

Information theory is the study of communication systems concerned with principles governing understanding, control, and predictability in communication. Information theory is related to and explains the transmission of information from a source to a final destination.

The message (what is being communicated) begins from the source, which can have a variety of origins—physical environment, learning resources, the health educator, or the individual's own thought processes—is transmitted in words or visual form; is picked up by a communication channel such as radio, television, or newspaper; reaches the receiver; and is then interpreted and used. For a clearer understanding and application of the theory to health education see Bedworth and Bedworth (1992, pp. 382-384).

Informed Consent

Informed consent is a legal tenet that holds providers responsible for ensuring that consumers or patients understand the risk and benefits of a procedure before it is administered.

Research participants must also be made aware of the nature of the research, its benefits, its risks, and the confidentiality of the data to be collected, before deciding whether or not to participate. Informed consent rules are intended to protect subjects, or participants, of research. For ethical and moral reasons, health educators need to have informed consent from subjects when carrying out research that involves humans.

Informed consent procedures are usually reviewed by institutional review boards (IRBs), which are part of major educational institutions, hospitals, and research institutions. A consent form created by the researcher must generally be read and signed by prospective research participants (Kramer, 1988; Powers & Knapp, 1990).

Injury Prevention

Injury prevention, now a public health issue, refers to efforts to reduce the risk of injuries before they happen. Passive approaches to injury prevention include childproof caps on bottles, and air bags and automatic seat belt restraints in automobiles. Active behavioral approaches include promoting seat belt and bicycle helmet use.

Innovation-Diffusion Theory

Innovation-diffusion theory identifies the process by which an innovation (new program) spreads through society. This theory is useful to health promotion because different social groups may comprehend things differently. Different people identify with and accept innovations differently, which plays an important role in the implementation and success of a program.

Innovation-diffusion theory helps explain how innovations spread from one person to another, one group to another, or in populations, and how innovations are adopted. The theory describes patterns target populations follow in adopting a program (Bunton & Macdonald, 1992; McKenzie & Jurs, 1993).

In-Service Training

In-service training is educational programs for advanced training or review training for persons in professions and on the job.

Example: A workshop for health educators on the job can inform or educate them on a current issue pertinent to their job, but of which they may be unaware.

Instructional Aid

Instructional aids are written or audiovisual materials used to implement a lesson plan or health promotion presentation.

Internal Validity

Internal validity is the degree to which an investigator's conclusions correctly describe what actually happened in a study. It is "the degree to which an observed change in an impact (behavior) or outcome (health status) rate (A) among individuals at risk (B) can be attributed to an intervention (C), Did C cause A to change among B?" (Windsor et al., 1994, pp. 14-15). The degree of certainty that a program caused the change that is being measured or the results of an evaluation is the internal validity. A study is said to have internal validity when the variables are logically consistent and represent a testable "causal relationship" (Oyster, Hanten, & Llorens, 1987; Vogt, 1993).

See **Validity.**

Internality-Externality Hypothesis of Obesity

The internality-externality hypothesis of obesity is a psychological theory proposing that obese people are more responsive to external cues, such as the presence of food or time of day, whereas non-obese people use more internal cues, such as hunger, to guide eating.

According to this theory, obese people confronted with an array of palatable-looking foods respond more readily to partaking of these foods and eat more than the nonobese, especially if the food is tasty and tempting.

This responsiveness, however, may be related to habits of dieting that obese people develop, a constant on-and-off dieting and refraining from dieting. This idea was put forward by Herman and Polivy (1980) and Rodin (1980) from observations showing that the responsiveness did not decrease when an obese person lost weight.

Intervention

An intervention is a planned, systematically applied combination of program elements, including procedures and methods designed to produce behavior changes or improve health status among individuals or a population at risk.

To carry out an intervention, health educators develop instruments such as questionnaires or review existing instruments for readability, ease of comprehension, sensitivity, and validity. This is done prior to the actual implementation of a program and forms part of the basis for program design. Types of interventions may include smoking cessation, exercise classes, and breast self-examination.

I

Intrinsic Motivation

Intrinsic motivation is displayed when a person engages in action or behavior for its own sake or reward. Often contrasted with extrinsic motivation, intrinsic motivation emphasizes performing a behavior for its own sake rather than for any external reward.

Example: People who exercise because they enjoy the activity in and of itself (intrinsic motivation) are more likely to continue to exercise than people who exercise because they expect to be rewarded (extrinsic motivation).

See **Extrinsic Motivation.**

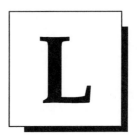

Learner Objective

Learner objectives, also called *instructional objectives* or *educational objectives,* are brief, clear statements that describe instructional intent in terms of the desired learning outcomes. They are written in three domains: cognitive (knowledge, comprehension), affective (emotional concepts such as interests and attitudes), and psychomotor (motor skills). Learner objectives are stated for individuals and begin with an action verb that is measurable.

Example: At the end of this session, the student will be able to state the key determinants of health behavior change.

See **Affective Domain, Cognitive Domain, Educational Objective,** and **Psychomotor Domain.**

Learner-Centered Guide

A learner-centered guide is a written document that describes what learners will be doing to achieve their objectives.

Lesson Plan

A lesson plan is a document delineating an active educational process in which a learner participates to reach educational goals. A lesson plan is an organizational structure in teaching that is built around the ordering of concepts, objectives, learning opportunities, and evaluation procedures within a specific lesson. A lesson plan is also called an instructional guide.

Example: The following lesson plan is one of a unit of lessons for a program titled Prevention of Alcoholism in the Workplace, covering a range of topics on alcoholism in the workplace.

Summary Outline

Title of Unit: Prevention of Alcoholism in the Workplace
Title of Session: Causes and Effects of Alcoholism in the Workplace
Learner Characteristics:
Age: 35 to 65
Sex: 65% male, 35% female employees
Ethnicity: 80% white, 20% other
Socioeconomic Status: Middle income level
Educational Level: 12 to 16 years of education
Educational Goals:

The goals of this session (lesson) are to:

1. Increase awareness of alcoholism in the workplace
2. Examine factors contributing to heavy alcohol intake at work
3. Increase knowledge of the adverse effects of alcohol on the individual and the business

Educational Concepts:

1. A large number of workers are using alcohol on the job at the workplace.
2. A number of factors contribute to alcohol use at work, including stress, working conditions, availability, and family problems.
3. Businesses are losing millions of dollars annually because of alcohol abuse on the job.

Lesson Plan

Educational Objectives:
At the end of this session, the learner will be able to:

1. Describe the prevalence of alcohol use in the workplace
2. List four factors contributing to heavy alcohol use at the workplace
3. Explain how alcoholism at the workplace leads to financial losses for business

Instructional Aids:
Handouts (alcohol related)
Overhead transparencies
Video

Teaching Time Required: 20 minutes for presentation, 30 minutes for discussion and activities

Time	Content	Method
5 minutes	Introduction/objectives	
15 minutes	Causes/effects	Lecture/transparencies
10 minutes	Alcoholism	Video
20 minutes	Causes/effects	Questions/discussions

Evaluation:

Participants' evaluation form, at end of lesson

Outline of Content:

1. Introduction (get acquainted)
   a. State objectives
   b. Define alcoholism and workplace
2. Prevalence of alcohol use at the workplace
   a. Results of surveys
   b. Demographics—age, education, gender
3. Causes of heavy alcohol use at the workplace
   a. Stress, frustration, boredom
   b. Availability of alcohol
   c. Family problems
   d. Social pressures

L

e. Work conditions
4. Effects of alcoholism on work and person
   a. Dollars lost annually
   b. Decreased productivity
   c. Increased absenteeism and sick leave
5. Video presentation
6. Question/answer/discussion period

Lewin's Field Theory

Lewin's field theory proposes that existing forces within a group influence one another. The theory teaches that behavior results from interactions between change or driving forces that pressure a group to move toward a goal, and resisting or restraining forces working to resist change. These forces tend to work against one another; when the resisting forces outweigh the driving forces no action is produced, because the behavior is blocked (Beach & Wise, 1980; Diamond, 1992; Kaufmann, 1973).

Field theory is important to health educators in that it helps to clarify why certain behaviors (health behaviors) are motivated and others are blocked (Butler, 1994; Ross & Mico, 1980).

To apply the theory, let individuals air their feelings regarding a certain issue requiring behavior change, and involve them in planning and problem solving to help identify resisting or restraining forces.

Example: In a smoking cessation program, knowledge of health risks involved in smoking and legislation restricting smoking are driving forces for change, but the pleasure one gets from smoking, peer pressure from smoking buddies, and fear of gaining weight after quitting can act as resisting forces. If these resisting forces outweigh the driving forces, the chances for positive behavior change are remote.

L

Lifestyle

The term *lifestyle* refers to a complex of related practices or constrained patterns of daily living maintained with some consistency in a person or group. Lifestyle involves cultural, physical, social, mental, spiritual, and environmental actions or characteristics of an individual or group (Grover, Gray, Joseph, Abrahamowicz, & Coupal, 1994; Moorhead, 1992; Sinha, 1992).

Lifestyle is "the culturally, socially, economically, and environmentally conditioned complex of actions characteristic of an individual, group, or community as a pattern of habituated behavior over time that is health related but not necessarily health directed" (Green & Kreuter, 1991, p. 433).

Lifestyle is a determining factor in the state of one's health, because the type of lifestyle one chooses may result in loss of health or premature death. Lifestyles that put people at risk include cigarette smoking, substance use and abuse (including alcohol and other drugs), poor nutritional habits, obesity, and a lack of exercise (Backett, Davison, & Mullen, 1994; Knutsen, 1994; Ornish et al., 1990).

Health education and promotion programs aim at changing lifestyles and behaviors that may put people at risk. However, health educators must keep in mind that individuals retain the right to make their own decisions regarding lifestyle choices.

Locus of Control

Locus of control is the perception of control over the environment, for example, the degree to which persons feel that they have control over their health outcomes. Health locus of control posits that health outcomes are determined either by an individual's actions or by external forces beyond one's control. Those with an internal locus of control believe that positive or negative events are under their personal control, whereas those with external control beliefs think that important outcomes are the result of luck, chance, or powerful others (Anderson, DeVellis, Sharpe, & Marcoux, 1994; Goodman, Cooley, Sewell, & Leavitt, 1994; Rotter, 1992).

Persons who feel that they are in control of their actions (internal locus of control) are more likely to believe that they can influence health outcomes; those who feel that outside or external forces in the environment (external locus of control) control their actions may be more likely to feel that health outcomes are also beyond their control.

Longitudinal Study

A longitudinal study is a research design in which the same individuals or groups are observed at different points in time over a designated period. A longitudinal study may involve a single cohort with similar characteristics, such as geographic area, a specified age range, race or ethnicity, marital status, and socioeconomic status, followed over time to investigate developments with respect to variables being tested.

Example: A group of children born from homes built near a toxic waste site may be studied at several points in time over a 15- to 20-year period for possible development of certain cancers.

L

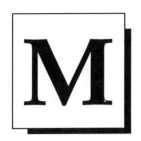

Method

In the health education field, methods are procedures used to determine what communication techniques and strategies should be employed to assist in the learning process. Methods include the use of media and different styles of teaching and learning, such as role playing, group instruction, class presentations, storytelling, and group discussion. Methods are systematic plans for implementing a program or project. The term is used interchangeably with *methodology*.

In research, the term is used to describe techniques, strategies, and other procedures. The methods or methodology section of the research design gives detailed information on the subject selection, instrumentation, whether a structured questionnaire was developed and pretested, contents of questionnaires, data collection procedures, and statistical analysis.

Model

A model is a conceptual basis for how a program or evaluation is supposed to work. A model is usually expressed graphically rather than textually, but may be in narrative form, explaining key factors and variables (Creswell, 1994). A model "serves to objectify and present a certain perspective or point of view about its nature and/or function" (Powers & Knapp, 1990, p. 88).

In public health, health promotion, and health education, a model may be necessary for several reasons. A model can help explain how behavior occurs, how health education is conducted, and how health education affects ongoing behavior. Models can describe resources and desired outcomes. Programs and evaluations are based on models, or theories, of human behavior (Windsor et al., 1994).

Example: A model can be used as a tool for setting up a health education program or research, for example, a program to lower fat intake in the diet. The model selected helps identify how people learn and the likelihood that the individuals from the target population will lower their fat intake in relation to certain factors or variables.

A model frequently used in health education is the Health Belief Model, to predict or explain health-related behavior based on people's perceptions and belief patterns.

See **Health Belief Model.**

Modeling

Modeling refers to a person's inclination to imitate another person's behavior. It is learning that takes place through observation of others and is an important process through which socialization occurs (Bandura, 1971, 1977; Bloomquist, 1986; Zimmerman & Rosenthal, 1974). Learning that takes place through modeling is more than just mimicking a behavior, and is very influential in helping to form behavior (Green et al., 1980). Modeling begins in early infancy and continues through adulthood; however, the strongest effects are during the early years of life. The effects of modeling can be both good and bad, depending on what is being modeled, and can play an important role in the promotion of healthful practices regarding alcohol, smoking, diet, and exercise.

M

Examples:

1. Much of the violence seen on television may be modeled by teenagers who have been influenced since early childhood through television viewing of violent scenes.

2. A child in a home in which both parents never smoked is more likely to model that behavior and never take up smoking during his or her lifetime.

Morbidity

Morbidity is a departure from a state of health and well-being, measured by numbers in a population who are ill, according to the type and duration of illness. Morbidity represents the number of persons living with a disease, expressed as a rate or proportion of persons with the disease to the total population.

Examples: The number of persons with AIDS, cancer, or heart disease in a given population.

Mores

Mores are strongly held norms or specific cultural expectations with a moral connotation. Mores are usually based on the values of a particular culture.

Mortality

Mortality represents the number of deaths that have occurred in a given time (e.g., within one year) or place (e.g., a specified population), and is usually expressed as a rate or proportion. Mortality statistics are important to public health and health promotion in planning preventive education programs for communities through providing information on causes of death and giving an indication of the risk of people dying from a particular disease during a definite period of time. Mortality data provide evidence of the frequency of a disease as it occurs in time, place, and persons, and may be important in predicting disease trends.

Multiple Causation

M

Multiple causation is a concept based on the idea that a given disease has a number of different causes: host-related factors linked to characteristics of the human population, agent-related factors associated with a specific cause, and environmental factors.

The idea underlying multiple causation is that disease, both infectious and chronic, is very complex and cannot be related to a single cause. To understand the process of a disease, one must look at a multiplicity of factors, including time and place.

Example: Heart disease cannot be related to one cause. There are several risk factors to be considered, including hypertension; family history of heart disease; social pressures; lack of exercise; cigarette smoking; obesity; and dietary excesses of salt, saturated fats, and cholesterol-laden foods.

M

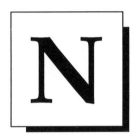

Needs Assessment

A needs assessment is a process of identifying problems and needs in a target population to make decisions, set priorities, set objectives, and explore alternative approaches or methods to aid in the planning and implementation of programs. Needs assessment is the study of the setting in which, for example, a health education program is to be conducted and is used largely in the first steps of planning.

Needs assessment involves making a social diagnosis to determine the social concerns of the people for whom the program is to be developed, an epidemiological diagnosis to review health statistics in an effort to decide on the most appropriate program to develop, a behavioral diagnosis to identify behavioral factors or barriers to health, an educational diagnosis to ascertain participants' knowledge of the issue and their health-related skills, and an administrative diagnosis to assess available resources necessary to achieve the program objectives (Butler, 1994; Green & Kreuter, 1991; Windsor et al., 1994).

Preparing a needs assessment is indispensable to program planning and may be the most critical step in the planning process. The process involves gathering data concerning the perceived health needs of the population to determine current and existing conditions; analyzing the data by looking at the incidence and prevalence of problems, including morality and morbidity statistics; and establishing priorities based on the ability to meet needs and available resources.

See **PRECEDE/PROCEED Model.**

Nominal Group Process

Nominal group process is a technique for generating and prioritizing needs or problems by asking group members to list problems in round robin fashion followed by rank ordering to determine the most pressing concerns.

N

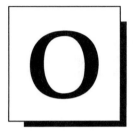

Objective

An objective is a precise statement of what we intend to accomplish, stating exactly where we are going and indicating how we will know when we have arrived. In health education, objectives are quantified statements of desired health status, specific activities to be completed, or health system performance to be achieved within a specified time period. Objectives are usually measurable and embody the aims or goals of an activity. Objectives include outcomes to be achieved, how they will be observed, and criteria for deciding whether or not they were achieved. Achievement is reflected in standards of performance and evaluation.

See **Behavioral Objective, Educational Objective,** and **Program Objective.**

Oral Rehydration Therapy

Oral rehydration therapy is a therapeutic solution of sodium concentrates, sugar, and water, used orally to prevent dehydration in children with diarrheal problems and concomitant vomiting. The most common components of the solution are sodium, potassium, and glucose. Oral rehydration therapy is most often used in international settings where physicians or nurses are not always readily available, and is the primary treatment for preventing death from dehydration. The solution can also be prepared at home (Banwell, 1990; Casteel & Fiedorek, 1990; Graeff et al., 1993; Sack, 1991).

Outcome Evaluation

Outcome evaluation is the assessment of the long-term effects of a program, for example, by observing health status and quality of life indicators in the earliest stages of a program and comparing them with the outcome. Outcome evaluation helps to determine whether or not the program met the stated goals (short and long term) and objectives (Green & Kreuter, 1991; Windsor et al., 1994). For example, outcome evaluation may ask, was there a reduction in maternal mortality rates in the target population as a result of the program?

Outcome evaluation is important to health educators because it helps to document the degree to which programs were conducted in accordance with the written plan, including goals, objectives, and results or benefits to participants.

See **Impact Evaluation** and **Program Evaluation.**

O

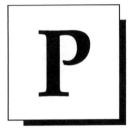

Paradigm

A paradigm is a broader concept than a theory (*see* **Theory**), and constitutes a way of looking at and interpreting the world, a particular field of study, a course of study, or problem under investigation. In health education, a paradigm is a model or framework that provides the context in which research is conducted and knowledge is accumulated.

Passive Smoking

Passive smoking is the inhalation of cigarette smoke by nonsmokers who are close to or in the same room with smokers or burning tobacco.

Patient Education

Patient education is any planned learning experience using a combination of teaching methods, counseling, and behavior modification techniques to influence the knowledge and health behavior of patients.

P

Patient education is concerned with helping patients learn how to care for themselves and to participate in decisions about their health care. It helps to prepare patients to deal with changes in medical care.

The greater part of patient education is done by nurses, although health educators and preventive medicine professionals are often employed to plan and teach patients about exercise regimens, dietary changes, and inherited traits of disease to help them reduce stress and cope with their illness or paralysis.

Performance Indicators

Performance indicators are a series of specific concepts and skills intended for 4th- 8th- and-11th grade students. They are intended to help health educators focus on the most essential knowledge and skills basic to the development of health-literate students. They also are intended to serve as a blueprint for organizing student assessment.

See **Health Education Standards.**

Physical Education

Physical education focuses on physical activity, fitness, and wellness in individuals, groups, communities, schools, and colleges. Physical education includes movement skills, knowledge, self-image, social development and interaction, and individual excellence. Physical education involves teaching strategies to promote confidence, self-assessment, cooperation, and independent learning.

Pilot Testing

Pilot testing is a method of checking out research intervention and methodology or health education programs and projects for the existence of unforeseen technical problems before the actual program or research project is launched.

A pilot test may refer to a test of a data collection instrument on a small test group as similar as possible to the group on which the instrument will actually be used. The pilot test enables the researcher to assess the clarity, sequence, length, and appropriateness of the instrument.

Pilot tests are designed to study data, collect information, and test an instrument (questionnaire) during the development phase of a research or intervention (program) to improve and document feasibility of program implementation; behavioral impact; and

P

appropriateness of content, methods, materials, or instruments. Pilot testing is an intervention measurement method for a health education and promotion program that is tried in the field. Data collected are used to revise and improve the intervention.

Example: Prior to conducting research, when a questionnaire is developed, a few copies (up to 50 depending on proposed sample size) are sent to a sample of people with the same characteristics as the intended research population. Responses enable a review of questionnaire for appropriateness.

Planned Approach to Community Health (PATCH)

Planned Approach to Community Health (PATCH) is a program developed by the Centers for Disease Control and Prevention (CDC) in 1983 as a model to guide community organizers in the development and implementation of health promotion. The program was designed to help communities analyze their needs and plan, implement, and evaluate health promotion programs. Currently, CDC provides technical assistance and training to states instead of communities. The approach is to begin at the grassroots level, such as a small group of people in a community who are interested in improving the overall health of community members. Using a team approach, people in the community make the decisions and do the work, with technical assistance from state or local health departments and the CDC. PATCH has its foundation in the diagnostic planning principles of the PRECEDE/PROCEED model and is aimed at translating complex methods of health education practice and intervention to communities and community organizations through health agencies. Training for PATCH is at the community level with collaborative efforts.

See **Centers for Disease Control and Prevention (CDC), Community Organization,** and **PRECEDE/PROCEED Model.**

Policy

A policy is a set of objectives or course of action considered advantageous or expedient in guiding the activities of an organization and providing authority for allocation of resources. Depending upon the organization or level of employment, health educators may not be actively involved in policy making, but may significantly influence policymakers. Health educators should, whenever possible, participate in policy development regarding health issues.

Policy Intervention

Policy intervention refers to those laws, policies, regulations, and formal and informal rules and understandings that are adopted on a collective basis to guide individual and collective behavior. It is the utilization of policy regulations to address problems and bring about change (Wallack, Dorfman, Jernigan, & Themba, 1993).

Population at Risk

A population at risk are those people who might have been exposed to a disease or other health problem, whether or not they become affected.

Population Attributable Risk

Population attributable risk is the number of excess cases of people with a disease in a population that can be attributed to a particular risk factor. The population attributable risk is a joint function of relative risk, the prevalence of a risk factor in the population, and the absolute risk of disease.

Example: Roughly 135,000 people die each year from lung cancer in the United States. The relative risk of lung cancer in smokers is 10 to 1; one third of the population smokes, so 101,000 lung cancer deaths per year are attributable to smoking behavior. Alternatively, there might have been 101,000 fewer deaths if no one smoked.

Postsecondary Health Education Program

"A post-secondary health education program is a planned set of health education policies, procedures, activities, and services that are directed to students, faculty and/or staff of colleges, universities, and other higher education institutions" (1990 Joint Committee on Health Education Terminology, 1991, p. 107). Health education at this level may include some general health courses for students, health promotion activities targeting employees and students, health services, and appropriate preparation of health educators and other professionals.

P

Posttest

A posttest in the health education field is an evaluation instrument that provides the educator with data that are interpreted in terms of the learning that is assumed to have taken place over a given period of time. It measures learning progress or behavior change over a given period.

PRECEDE/PROCEED Model

The PRECEDE/PROCEED model describes five steps in planning and evaluating a health promotion program:

1. The social diagnosis (assessment of quality of life)
2. An epidemiological diagnosis (use of epidemiological data to determine health problems)
3. Behavioral diagnosis (identifying health-related and non-health-related behaviors)
4. Educational diagnosis (sorting factors that may potentially affect health behaviors)
5. Administrative diagnosis (actual development and implementation of program)

The acronym PRECEDE stands for the diagnostic phases of health education and promotion planning: predisposing, reinforcing, and enabling constructs in educational diagnosis and evaluation. This framework also helps health planners to identify priorities and set objectives for program implementation and evaluation and include factors involved in implementation, which is referred to as PROCEED: policy, regulatory, and organizational constructs in educational and environmental development (Bates & Winder, 1984; Green & Kreuter, 1991; Green et al., 1980; Kunstel, 1978).

This model is of particular importance to health educators as it forces them to deal with realities and recognize theories of behavior change in conducting health behavior change programs.

Predictable Variable

In considering the association between cause and effect, the variable that precedes the other (or is presumed on biologic grounds to be antecedent) is called the predictable variable.

Example: In the relationship between gender and occurrence of heart disease, gender is the predictor variable.

Predisposing Factor

Predisposing factors are independent constructs such as knowledge, attitudes, beliefs, values, and perceptions in a person or population that facilitate or hinder motivation for change. These characteristics are considered antecedents to the occurrence of particular health-related behaviors (Green & Kreuter, 1991; Green et al., 1980; Valente, Sobal, Muncie, Levine, & Antilitz, 1986).

Example: If an AIDS prevention education program is being planned for teenagers, predisposing factors that may be considered are teenagers' knowledge about AIDS, attitudes toward behavior that put them at risk, beliefs about how the disease is transmitted, and their perception of themselves as being invincible.

Preferred Provider Organization (PPO)

The preferred provider organization (PPO) is a managed care arrangement to deliver health services with a fixed discounted fee for service under specific terms of agreement. Hospitals or other caregivers contract to provide health services to a designated group of consumers. Outpatient services are provided, as well as primary intervention, and prevention is promoted through health education strategies.

PPOs started as a response to the demand for lower health care cost. Individuals under this plan may have little or no deductible. Practicing physicians may or may not practice in the same location (de Lissovoy, Rice, Gabel, & Gelzer, 1987; Mielke, 1994).

See **Health Maintenance Organization (HMO).**

Pretest

A pretest is a process in formative research or designing a program of systematically gathering target audience reactions to messages and materials before they are produced in final form, or measuring a variable before an intervention begins. Various techniques are used to determine, for example, relevance of program to audience; relevance of a questionnaire to intended target group; or level of existing knowledge of topic prior to a presentation, lecture, workshop, or course of study. The pretest is administered before the program, experiment, or research.

Prevalence

Prevalence is a measure of the extent of a health problem or disease in a population based on the total number (old and new) of existing cases in a population at a given time. From a public health perspective, prevalence is of great importance, because health care services may be distributed according to the existing health and disease status of the population (Kramer, 1988).

Prevention

In the health field, prevention is the process whereby specific action is taken to prevent or reduce the possibility of a health problem or condition developing and to minimize any damage that may have resulted from a previous condition.

There are three levels of prevention: primary (stopping the disease before it occurs), secondary (early detection and prompt treatment to deter further decay), and tertiary (interventions to limit further disability and early death).

See **Primary Prevention, Secondary Prevention,** and **Tertiary Prevention.**

Preventive Services

Preventive services primarily involve interventions provided in clinical settings, but are not limited to these settings. Among the current priority areas are maternal and infant health, cancer, heart disease and stroke, HIV infection, sexually transmitted diseases (STDs), and immunization for infectious diseases.

Preventive services may involve early prenatal care to prevent babies with low birth weight and infant deaths; reduction of tobacco use, dietary fat intake, and high blood pressure, in an effort to prevent heart disease and stroke; mammography, clinical breast examination, Pap tests, fecal occult blood tests, and digital rectal examinations to detect and treat cancers before they spread; increasing use of condoms among sexually active men with multiple partners to prevent STDs; and increasing immunization to help eliminate infectious diseases such as tuberculosis, diphtheria, polio, rubella, and measles.

P

Primary Health Care

Primary health care is the first level of contact for individuals, family, and community to obtain basic health care that does not necessarily require a physician. It is essential health care provided to communities by means acceptable to them, with their participation, and at an affordable cost.

Primary health care includes health education, environmental sanitation (particularly food and water), promotion of nutrition, maternal and child health programs, immunization, family planning, and appropriate treatment of common diseases and injuries. Primary health care, mostly seen in developing countries and poorer nations, is usually an integral part of the country's health care system. In setting up a primary health care program, goals are developed, budgets identified and assigned, strategies formulated, and pilot projects undertaken (Carlaw & Ward, 1988).

Personnel for primary health care are auxiliary workers; health educators; dental hygienists; nurses; midwives; nurse practitioners; village health workers; and occasionally, a physician or dentist (Bossert & Parker, 1984). Primary health care may vary from country to country depending on needs and resources.

Example: In 1981, Haiti established a primary health care program in a rural area to serve 115,000 persons. The Albert Schweitzer Hospital extended community-based services to help reduce tetanus, malnutrition, tuberculosis, and diarrhea, diseases that accounted for use of a high percentage of hospital beds. Preventive services included health education in the areas of nutrition, sanitation, oral rehydration therapy (see Oral Rehydration Therapy), and immunization, as well as support for traditional birth attendants. The staff comprised 2 physicians, 2 nurses, 30 auxiliaries (support personnel), and a sanitary officer (Basch, 1990). One of the aims of this program was to free hospital beds for more threatening health problems.

Primary Prevention

Primary prevention is the intervention or use of specific strategies and programs to reduce the occurrence of disease in a population. The first level of prevention, it is aimed at deterring disease before it occurs (Bates & Winder, 1984; Butler, 1994; Fox, Hall, & Elveback, 1970).

P

Much of primary prevention is accomplished through health promotion and education, and certain environmental protection actions. Interventions may include water fluoridation to prevent dental decay, eradication of mosquitoes to prevent malaria, promoting sexual abstinence among teenagers to prevent HIV/AIDS transmission, and the wearing of safety equipment to prevent accidents when working with machinery.

Private Health Agency

A private health agency is a nongovernmental agency organized as a profit or nonprofit incorporated (voluntary), unincorporated (voluntary), or commercial organization concerned with health, health services, and health education on primary, secondary, and tertiary levels of prevention.

Examples: American Heart Association, National Dairy Council.
See **Voluntary Health Organization** or **Agency.**

PROCEED

PROCEED, the acronym for *p*olicy, *r*egulatory, and *o*rganizational *c*onstructs in *e*ducational and *e*nvironmental *d*evelopment, is a theoretical model used in the developmental phase of health education program planning. It follows the diagnostic phase, providing additional measures for developing policy and initiating the implementation and evaluation process of a health program (Green & Kreuter, 1991).
See **PRECEDE/PROCEED Model.**

Process Evaluation

Process evaluation is used to study program implementation to detect problems early on and determine whether the program strayed from the protocol. Assessing the materials used, program personnel performance, quality of professional practice, and services through observation or periodic surveys assists in making changes or adjustments for successful completion of the program.

Process evaluation is an ongoing examination of what is delivered and how it is delivered and includes program conception, program staff, methods, activities, and effectiveness and efficiency in reaching the target group or population.

Process evaluation is "designed to document the degree to which program procedures were conducted according to a written program plan: How much of the intervention was provided, to whom, when, and by whom?" (Windsor et al., 1994, p. 14).
See **Evaluation** and **Program Evaluation.**

Program Evaluation

Program evaluation is an appraisal of a program to demonstrate its worth or effectiveness and to make recommendation for improvements. Program evaluation helps in making comparisons with different types of programs, looking at achievements; cost-effectiveness; appropriateness; and, if funded, whether requirements for funding were met (Green et al., 1980; Weiss, 1972; Windsor et al., 1994). The term *assessment* is also used for program evaluation.
See **Evaluation.**

Program Implementation

Program implementation is the execution or actual carrying out of a planned program, when decisions are put into actions.

Program Objective

A program objective is a specific measurable statement of a desired program outcome. Program objectives should be realistic and consistent with the policies and procedures of the organization or community agency sponsoring the program.

Example: By the end of the program, participants will be able to list evaluation methodologies appropriate to health education programs.

Program Planning

Program planning is the process in which needs (real or perceived) are assessed, identified, analyzed, and defined; problems are diagnosed; resources are allocated; and barriers are assessed in order to achieve objectives. Then a program or plan of solution is designed based on the needs assessment. The PRECEDE/PROCEED model can be used.

In the health education field, program planning begins with an interest in a specific health issue, and is concerned with the group at risk, incidence and prevalence rates, specific behaviors to be targeted, and how these may change or be addressed with a health education intervention. Program planning is also concerned with resources (materials, personnel, money, time) that are available or can be made available to put the intervention into effect (Delbecq, 1974; Green & Kreuter, 1991; Windsor et al., 1994).

Health educators and promoters are usually employed by agencies or organizations to develop or plan health-related programs. This involves the design, implementation, and evaluation of a program plan suited to what the organization wants, what consumers need, and what is beneficial and cost-effective to both.

Psychomotor Domain

The psychomotor domain concerns learning that applies knowledge to life situations and involves neuromuscular coordination, including physical skills, habits developed, and general practices.

Example: Individuals develop appropriate health behavior patterns such as an annual Pap test, annual physical or dental examination, or routine breast self-examination.

Learning objectives may also be stated in the psychomotor domain.

Example: In a hypertension prevention program being offered to adult women, one of the activities included the use of a home monitoring kit to monitor their blood pressure. Objectives in the psychomotor domain are (a) by the end of this session, participants will be able to take their blood pressure accurately under the supervision of the health educator; or (b) at the end of this session, each participant will be able to operate the blood pressure measuring equipment.

Psychosomatic Illness

Psychosomatic illness consists of bodily symptoms resulting from mental conflict instead of a physiological basis. There is clearly a mind-body disease relationship, but this is mainly due to personality. People may think they are sick and may even show symptoms, but tests reveal that there is nothing physiologically wrong. It is estimated that nearly 50% of people seeking medical attention suffer from some psychosomatic disorder associated with emotional stress

(Bedworth & Bedworth, 1992). Health education and promotion endeavors should consider this factor in approaches to help people.

Public Health

Public health is the science and art of preventing disease, prolonging life, and promoting health and efficiency through organized community effort for the sanitation of the environment, control of communicable infections, education in personal hygiene, organization of medical and nursing services, and the development of the social machinery to ensure everyone a standard of living adequate for the maintenance of health (Bunton & Macdonald, 1992; Rubinson & Alles, 1984; Winslow, 1920).

Public health focuses primarily on the health of populations, communities, and organizations rather than individuals, and is committed to social responsibility. Usually, public health is concerned with a health problem, based on the assumption that the social, physical, and political environments play major roles in the amelioration of the problem (Hanlon & Pickett, 1984; Lee & Estes, 1990).

Public health, a major force in keeping the nation well, recognizes personal health habits as a strong influence in the causes of morbidity and mortality. The key components of public health include, but are not limited to, health policy, epidemiology, nutrition, occupational and environmental health, health education, control of communicable disease, health services administration, and injury control. Public health is also devoted to primary prevention (avoiding disease before it occurs).

Public Service Announcements

Public service announcements are messages intended for the public disseminated without charge by the media (print, television, radio). This service is regularly used by health educators and other health professionals for getting health-related messages to the public.

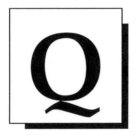

Qualitative Approach

A qualitative approach is a research method that employs descriptive methodology to collect data such as interviews, case studies, focus groups, and observations. It is a more naturalistic approach than the traditional quantitative approach to research (Steckler, McLeroy, Goodman, Bird, & McCormick, 1992; Windsor et al., 1994).

Qualitative approach is an inquiry process of understanding social or human problems, usually conducted in a natural setting and including the reporting of informants' views. Using the qualitative approach, investigators interact with their study subjects, sometimes living with them in the community, and observing them over a period of time. Facts are then reported from evidence gathered. The style used to report the findings may be different from that of traditional research, less formal, more personal, and based on terms that emerge during the study.

See **Quantitative Approach.**

Quality Assurance

Quality assurance is a formal process of assessing the quality of a program or project, and making improvements to assure providers, financiers such as funding agencies, and consumers that professional activities have been performed appropriately. Quality assurance, as defined by Windsor and colleagues (1994), is "the appropriateness of a set of professional procedures for a problem and objectives to be achieved" (p. 101).

Quality assurance consists of observing and assessing program procedures, including how the staff carries out the program. A quality assurance investigator examines events that took place, such as problems that arose during program development and implementation, and demands proper documentation of the competence of key personnel or providers (Rubinson & Alles, 1984).

Quality of Life

Quality of life is people's perception whether or not their needs are being satisfied and opportunities presented that allow for achievement of happiness and fulfillment. It is used as a public health measure ("Quality of Life," 1994).

In the PRECEDE framework of planning, the social diagnosis is concerned with the assessment of quality of life of community members, and looks at social indicators (e.g., unemployment rate, overcrowding, and housing conditions). Major concerns of the population are gathered and used in the analysis of health problems and program planning (Green & Kreuter, 1991).

The assessment of quality of life helps health professionals to understand the situation through the eyes of community members, the perceptions they have of quality of life, and what is important to them. Health promotion and education are aimed at improving quality of life through the promotion of healthy conditions, but to be effective these conditions must be viewed as important by community members.

Quality of life may be assessed through simple questionnaires, face-to-face interviews, or focus groups or forums to obtain a consensus as to priorities. Discussions are important because even in the same community people may have different perceptions on quality of life concerns related to different cultural backgrounds, interests, and felt needs.

See **PRECEDE/PROCEED Model** and **Social Diagnosis.**

Q

Quantitative Approach

A quantitative approach is a deductive method (applying a generally accepted principle to an individual case) that employs hard data, such as counts, ratings, scores, or classifications, to summarize findings.

The quantitative approach to research, as opposed to the qualitative method, is based on the testing of a theory composed of variables. Quantitative research involves measurements with numbers, statistical procedures, and data analysis, in order to determine whether or not the predictions of a theory or hypothesis are true.

The quantitative method is a more traditional approach to research than qualitative approaches. The researcher remains distant from and independent of the subjects being studied, controls for bias, selects systematic samples, and tests hypotheses (chosen prior to the study) to determine cause and effect. The quantitative approach helps researchers to develop certain generalizations (which contribute to theories) and enables them to predict and explain results (Creswell, 1994; Windsor et al., 1994).

See **Qualitative Approach.**

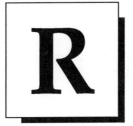

Reciprocal Determinism

Reciprocal determinism is the concept that there is an interaction among the individual, the behavior, and the environment in reference to behavior changes—that the environment can shape a person and the person can shape the environment. In Bandura's (1977) social cognitive theory, reciprocal determinism is the continuous shared interaction among a person's behavior, personality, and environment.

See **Social Cognitive Theory.**

Reinforcing Factor

A reinforcing factor is a reward, feedback, or incentive that a learner receives from others subsequent to the adoption of a behavior—in the context of the health education field, a health behavior. Reinforcing factors contribute to the individual's persistence in the behavior and serve to strengthen the motivation. Reinforcing factors can include attitudes and behavior of health personnel, peers, employees, parents, and relatives.

Relapse Prevention

Relapse prevention is any maintenance strategy used to prevent an individual from reverting to behaviors after recent lifestyle modification or behavior change. A program for relapse prevention uses self-control principles to help individuals cope with problems in the process of changing behavior (Marlatt & Gordon, 1985; Shumaker, Schron, & Ockerie, 1990).

R

Example: A person attends a smoking cessation seminar and quits smoking, but he or she may slip back into the smoking habit if not provided with a maintenance program.

Relative Risk

Relative risk is the ratio of the incidence or chance of a disease or health problem in individuals exposed to a risk factor compared with the risk of disease or health in individuals without exposure.

Example: The relative risk of lung cancer for a 40-year-old heavy cigarette smoker compared with a nonsmoker is about 10 to 1, and the relative risk of heart disease is about 2 to 1.

Reliability

Reliability is a term used in research for consistency in the measurement process of information or research results if the study or experiment is repeated. If an instrument (questionnaire) is reliable, it will give the same (or almost the same) results, but not perfect accuracy, every time it is used.

Resiliency

Resiliency is a fairly new term for factors that contribute to survival and decisions related to health-promoting choices, especially in cases of individuals who display several risk factors that make healthy choices unlikely.

Retroactive Facilitation

Retroactive facilitation is the review of material or the discovery of new explicit relationships resulting in greater retention of a previous experience.

Retroactive Inhibition

Retroactive inhibition refers to the effect that present learning can have on the retention of previously learned material. New learning, or accumulation of facts about a basic food group, for example, may hinder the retention of previous learning about that food group, especially if there is some confusion about previous information.

Risk Behavior

Risk behaviors are practices, habits, or actions that put individuals at risk for disease or health-related problems, including cigarette smoking, sexual intercourse at an early age, multiple sex partners, consumption of high-fat foods, driving without seat belts, bicycle or motorcycle riding without a helmet, drug use, and physical fights (Grunbaum & Basen-Engquist, 1993; "Quality of Life," 1994; Zimmerman & Olson, 1994).

Risk Factor

Risk factors are factors such as social, environmental, and lifestyle or behavioral causes known to be associated with an individual's increasing risk or probability of acquiring a specific disease.

Risk Reduction

Risk reduction is the reduction of factors that put individuals at risk of developing a health problem or a disease.

See **Risk Factors.**

Role Delineation

Role delineation is the process of clarifying the role performed by health educators through the specification of responsibilities and functions and the identification of requisite skills and knowledge.

See **Entry-Level Health Educator.**

R

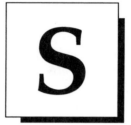

Sampling

Sampling is the process by which a portion of a population is selected for study where the goal is to represent the target population as closely as possible and minimize bias due to selection. It is the selection of a few observations to serve as the basis for arriving at general conclusions (Kish, 1987).

Sampling is necessary to overcome the problem of representativeness. Selecting people (e.g., teenagers attending a sexually transmitted disease, or STD, clinic) randomly or by a systematic method (e.g., every fifth teenager who visits the clinic) gives a basis for expecting the data to be representative of the population as a whole.

When an evaluation or survey research is being planned, one of the first concerns is the sample size and its selection. In selecting a sample, some random component should be included in order to generalize to the population being studied. One may select a simple random, systematic, clustered, or stratified sampling technique.

Example: To select a systematic random sample, divide the population (e.g., 40,000) by the desired sample size (e.g., 400), which results in a sampling interval of 100. From the 40,000, select every 100th name, and 400 cases will be systematically obtained. To include the random component, select a random starting number (from a random table available in most statistics books) between 1 and 100. Starting with that case, select every 100th name. Thus if the starting number is 57, then select every 100th number (157, 257, 357, etc.) until 400 cases are selected for the study. If the population is recorded in alphabetical order, the sampling is considered unbiased, adding strength to the interpretation of the data.

School-Based Health Services

School-based health services are support services based at the school to ensure access to health care for students. These services may include health clinics, child care (for teen parents to continue their education), and appropriate social and health services. School-based health services may also include violence prevention; weight reduction, nutrition, and other health education services; acute care; laboratory services; health-screening examinations; and psychosocial services (Taras, 1994; Yates, 1994).

School Health

School health involves a multiphasic program covering the physiological, sociological, psychological, and spiritual aspects of health in a school setting.

School health is concerned with health education (both formal and informal), instruction (a program of planned activities that takes place in the school), health services (rendered by a nurse or other health professionals), and healthful school environment (safe and healthful climate and surroundings). School health is important because the health status of the students may affect their learning and ability to achieve; such effects can be negative or positive. Schools are thought of as institutions that must offer support, be responsible for the children's health, and provide educational opportunity to help students live and adjust to society. Schools have a unique opportunity to promote health and aid in the prevention of disease (Belzer & McIntyre, 1994; Cornacchia, Olsen, & Nickerson, 1991).

School Health Education

School health education is that component of the total school health program (health services, healthful school environment, health instruction) that provides teaching and learning experiences. School health education is also concerned with developing, implementing, and evaluating planned instructional programs and activities that favorably influence knowledge, attitudes, habits, practices, appreciations, and conduct pertaining to the health of students. School health education is aimed at protecting and promoting the well-being of students and school personnel. It is usually planned and conducted under the supervision of school personnel and with involvement of community health personnel (Hamburg, 1993; Redican, Olsen, & Baffi, 1986; Schall, 1994).

See **Healthful School Environment, School Health Environment, School Health Instruction,** and **School Health Environment.**

School Health Educator

A school health educator is a person with professional preparation in the field of school health education who meets the teaching requirements of his or her state and shows competence in developing, delivering, and evaluating curricula that will help to enhance health knowledge, attitudes, and problem-solving skills for students and adults in the school setting.

School Health Environment

The school health environment is an important component of comprehensive school health education concerned with establishing a safe climate for children that enhances opportunities for learning. It includes site selection (away from landfills), school design, number of rest rooms, type of building, safe playgrounds, acceptable water supply, and other environmental concerns (Anderson & Creswell, 1980; Rudd & Walsh, 1993).

See **Healthful School Environment** and **School Health.**

School Health Instruction

School health instruction begins in preschool with a variety of content areas, such as personal health and hygiene, substance use and abuse, safety and accident prevention, family life, nutrition education, growth and development, disease prevention and control, and environmental health. Instructional methods must be appropriate to behavior change and outcome oriented.

See **School Health Education.**

School Health Services

School health services are procedures to promote, appraise, and protect the health of schoolchildren. Services may be provided by physicians, nurses, teachers, dentists, dietitians, school counselors, and others (Anderson & Creswell, 1980; Brandon, 1993; Yates, 1994).

School health services provide first aid and care for those who may become injured or ill at school; immunization; and screening for dental caries, sickle cell anemia, and other conditions.

"School health services are that part of the school health program provided by physicians, nurses, dentists, health educators, other allied health personnel, social workers, teachers and others to appraise, protect and promote the health of students and school personnel. These services are designed to insure access to and the appropriate use of primary health care services, prevent and control communicable disease, provide emergency care for injury or sudden illness, promote and provide optimum sanitary conditions in a safe school facility and environment, and provide concurrent learning opportunities which are conducive to the maintenance and promotion of individual and community health" (1990 Joint Committee on Health Education Terminology, 1991, p. 106).

See **School Health.**

Secondary Prevention

Secondary prevention is any intervention strategy, such as case finding, screening, and treatment, intended to reduce the presence of an existing disease in a population, thus preventing further deterioration and early death.

Secondary prevention is concerned with early detection and prompt treatment of disease. The goal is to identify the disease at its earliest stage and apply appropriate treatments to limit its severity.

Example: Detecting breast cancer in its earliest stage (before metastasis, or spread) and intervening with treatment (surgery and/or chemotherapy).

See **Prevention.**

Self-Efficacy

Based on Bandura's social cognitive theory, self-efficacy constitutes a person's belief in his or her ability to perform a specific behavior. Self-efficacy is a construct that refers to the internal state that a person experiences, such as competence or ability to perform a desired task or behavior (Bandura, 1982; Strecher, DeVellis, Becker, & Rosenstock, 1986).

Example: A typical statement of self-efficacy: How confident are you that you could perform Behavior X in Situation Y?
See **Social Cognitive Theory.**

Self-Management

Self-management is the concept that individuals can monitor a health behavior goal by keeping records of their own target behavior and factors associated with the behavior, and provide self-rewards or reinforcements that will help to increase the likelihood of achieving the goal. Self-management can be used in various health settings as part of a behavioral intervention strategy in health promotion programs.

Self-Regulation

Self-regulation is the act or process of controlling health-threatening behavior by active recall of long-term consequences of the behavior. One of the aims of health promotion is to enable individuals to take control over, or regulate, their behavior. This involves identifying cues in the environment or in the individual's own thoughts and feelings that can help in controlling, or regulating, behavior.

Sensitivity

Sensitivity, in the health field, is a measurement used to evaluate diagnostic, prognostic, and screening tests to determine how well a test can discriminate between the diseased and the nondiseased. Sensitivity refers to the proportion of subjects with a disease who have a positive test result. It indicates how good a test is at identifying cases of the disease in a population or group.
See **Specificity** and **Validity.**

Set Point Theory

According to set point theory, each person has an internally predetermined weight that the body attempts to maintain, despite efforts to change. The body's metabolism may even change to preserve the weight.

Set point theory was tested by Keys, Brozek, Henschel, Michelson, and Taylor (1950) in research involving men on a starvation diet whose bodies resisted losing weight. Other studies designed to help people gain or lose weight have showed similar effects (Keys et al., 1950). Personal set points may differ from societal ideal weights. An understanding of this theory is important to health educators when conducting programs designed to help individuals lose weight.

Sick-Role Behavior

Sick-role behavior is any activity undertaken for the purpose of getting well by persons who consider themselves to be ill or who were diagnosed with a medical problem (Mayou, 1984). Sick-role behavior is similar to illness behavior.

Example: Visiting a doctor for treatment and following the treatment protocol.

See **Illness Behavior.**

Social Cognitive Theory

Social cognitive (formerly called social learning) theory is a general model of behavior set forth by Bandura (1977, 1982) emphasizing the effect of the social environment and cognitive mediators such as beliefs on behavior, and the reciprocal effect of behavior on environment and cognition. Social cognitive theory explains learning as a reciprocal interaction among an individual's environment, thought processes, and behavior, so that learning takes place through synthesized thoughts.

Social cognitive theory is applicable to health promotion in explaining and predicting behavior through key concepts such as incentives and outcome expectations. According to social cognitive theory, change is a function of expectations; for example, expectations of what will be the results of participating in a behavior change activity, or expectations of one's ability to execute the behavior. Three key aspects to the theory are vicarious learning or imitation of the behavior, the use of symbols, and principles of self-management. The most prominent concept of the theory is self-efficacy (Rosenstock, Strecher, & Becker, 1988).

See **Self-Efficacy** and **Reciprocal Determinism.**

Social Comparison Theory

Social comparison theory is a social-psychological theory suggesting that when people are confused about their internal state, they turn to others in order to interpret the situation.

Social Diagnosis

Social diagnosis is a social needs assessment concerned with quality of life (training, reduced productivity, employment, and disability). The process utilizes multiple information-gathering activities designed to expand understanding of individual and community perceptions of needs, or quality of life, as defined by social problems such as unwed teenage pregnancies, violence, unemployment, job absenteeism, and crime (Bauer, 1966; Green et al., 1980; Kaplan, 1988).

Social diagnosis has also been described as the "process of determining people's perceptions of their own needs or quality of life, and their aspirations for the common good, through broad participation and the application of multiple information-gathering activities designed to expand understanding of the community" (Green & Kreuter, 1991, p. 45). In a social diagnosis, investigators look at problems defined for a population by economic and social indicators or by individuals in terms of their quality of life.

See **PRECEDE/PROCEED Model.**

Social Ecology Framework

Social ecology framework is a way of looking at how people interact with their physical, social, and cultural environments. Ecology, of course, refers to the study of relationships between an organism (any individual life form) and its environment. The social ecology approach involves the identification of physical and social characteristics of the environment that may affect a person's health. These characteristics may include stress influenced by change of residence, noise in the neighborhood, social isolation, access to health care facilities, and safety. A consideration of these factors may lead to the development of health promotion programs focusing on change (Kaplan et al., 1993).

Social ecology framework is useful to community health promotion, as it emphasizes the importance of environmental changes on health and can provide clues about the type of changes in the environment that facilitate healthful behaviors (Stokols, 1992).

Social Marketing Framework

Social marketing framework applies marketing principles and techniques to promote change in health behavior. The concept was developed by Philip Kotler (1982), and is based on the four Ps of marketing: product, promotion, place, and price.

Applied to health promotion, this concept requires program planners to determine the products and services that are acceptable to the community. Products may include vegetarian cookbooks or pamphlets with the basic food guide information. Services may include the development of nutrition education programs and cooking classes.

The promotion aspect of the health program can be accomplished through the media, distribution of flyers, personal invitations, and word of mouth. The right place must also be found to make the products and services available to the community. Services and products can be offered at community centers, service clubs, tribal halls, churches, and work sites. In addition, health education materials can be made available at supermarkets, public libraries, clinics, and hospital waiting rooms.

Price includes the cost to produce and market the products and services (health education programs), taking into consideration time, transportation opportunities, and accessibility.

Social Support

Social support is usually defined by the number of social contacts people maintain, such as family; friends; church members; or others one can rely on, care about, and love (Cobb, 1976). Social support includes the satisfaction that is felt with social relationships.

It is believed that social relationships have an effect upon health outcomes. A network of family, friends, and other social contacts may help to ease stress and tensions resulting from sickness or injuries (Porritt, 1979). According to Bellock and Breslow (1972), people who experience good social support also seem to have healthier lifestyles. Positive social relationships may enhance health and well-being and mental health outcomes, and have a protective effect for problems such as heart disease.

Building social support is a meaningful method of reinforcing self-directed health behaviors, and can be informal, for example, asking a friend or family member to exercise with you or be your

S

buddy during the course of a smoking cessation program (Fenlason & Beehr, 1994).

There are also more formal support groups for medical problems. Support groups initiated by the American Cancer Society for women who have undergone mastectomies or other treatment for breast cancer are one such example. These groups meet at scheduled times to offer support and learn more about the problem.

Specificity

Specificity is used to evaluate diagnostic, examination, and screening tests to determine how well a test can discriminate between the diseased and the nondiseased. Specificity refers to the proportion of subjects without the disease who have a negative test result. It indicates how good a test is at identifying people without the disease in question.

Specificity is a measure of validity and is often defined as the proportion without the disease or with a negative measure. Specificity and sensitivity are usually considered together as measures of validity.

See **Sensitivity** and **Validity.**

Stages of Change

Based on Prochaska and DiClemente's transtheoretical model, stages of change are the sequence of stages a person goes through when attempting to change a behavior: precontemplation, contemplation, decision, action, and maintenance. People seem to move through an orderly sequence of change, some more rapidly than others. At each stage of change, different processes of change, or intervention approaches, are needed (DiClemente et al., 1991; Kaplan et al., 1993).

In the precontemplation stage, people (precontemplators) have no intention to change a behavior, but will at least become aware of the problem or behavior. In the contemplation stage, people (now contemplators) are thinking about making a change and are reevaluating their behaviors. Then a decision is made. In the action stage, a person changes the behavior, and in the maintenance stage the behavior change is sustained.

See **Transtheoretical Model.**

Strategy

A strategy is a plan of action for achieving specific objectives, anticipating both barriers and resources.

Stress Response

Stress responses are relatively stereotypic sets of interacting psychological and biological patterns that organisms exhibit in response to exposure to a stressor. When the body experiences certain stressful events, a stress response is induced if the person feels that he or she cannot cope with the adversity or stressor (Kaplan et al., 1993).

Example: A stress response is created when a person adjusts to a stressor, such as death of a loved one or recent news of test results indicating disease such as cancer.

See **Stressor.**

Stress-Buffering Model

According to the stress-buffering model, social support absorbs the impact of stress. This model predicts that the relationship between social support and health outcome should occur only for those under high levels of stress, and describes the protective effects that social support has on an individual.

According to this model, "social support may intervene in the pathway between the stressful event and the receiver" (individual) (McMahon, Schram, & Davidson, 1993, p. 242). In other words, friends may intervene by encouraging the person who is experiencing the stress, and the more positive the response, the more effective should be the outcome (McMahon et al., 1993; Ulbrich & Bradsher, 1993).

The model also indicates that when there is high stress and low social support, the result can be illness; but when there is high stress and high social support, then the impact of stress is buffered or absorbed (DesCamp & Thomas, 1993; Revenson & Majerovitz, 1991).

See **Social Support.**

Stressor

A stressor is any stimulus that makes demands on an individual requiring adaptation (e.g., making beneficial alterations to one's living conditions) or adjustment (modifying or altering one's behavior) (Selye, 1976).

S

Summative Evaluation

A stressor may be an event, physical or environmental, that triggers a response or threatens a person's existence and well-being, and makes demands that require adaptation (Selye, 1978; Sheridan & Perkins, 1992; Vlisides, Eddy, & Mozie, 1994; Whitehead, 1994).

Examples: Very cold weather, lack of sleep, sustained physical exercise, excessive noise, sorrow (from death of a family member), joy (news that you just won big money), fear, and frustration.

Summative Evaluation

Summative evaluation occurs at the completion of a program in order to determine its effectiveness in achieving program objectives and whether the program should be continued. A summative evaluation also helps in measuring achievements, such as how many individuals actually changed a targeted behavior.

See **Impact Evaluation, Outcome Evaluation,** and **Program Evaluation.**

Surveillance

In the health field, surveillance is the process of monitoring diseases as they occur. It is the "continuing scrutiny of all aspects of occurrence and spread of disease that are pertinent to effective control" (Benenson, 1990, p. 507).

Example: The Centers for Disease Control and Prevention (CDC) are involved with surveillance of diseases and provide mortality and morbidity reports, reports of field investigations of epidemics, identification of infectious agents and new diseases, reports on effects of vaccines, information regarding immunity levels in population segments, and other relevant data. CDC surveillance summaries of diseases are published in the *Morbidity and Mortality Weekly Report* (MMWR).

Survey

A survey is a method of collecting data from a group or population to estimate the norms and distribution of characteristics from a sample. Surveys usually employ instruments such as questionnaires, interviews, or direct observation.

The purpose of a survey is to obtain specific information from a specified group of people or population. A survey can be conducted in a variety of formats, such as face-to-face interviews, mailed or telephone questionnaires, focus groups, or direct observation.

Survey results can be used as baseline data for measuring change, for delineating and describing problems in a population, and for adding to the body of knowledge on the subject or issue under consideration.

S

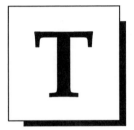

Target Group or Population

A target group is a set of people or a community being targeted or focused on, for example, for a prevention program aimed at reducing the incidence of disease or addressing some health condition.

Example: Children ages 1 through 5 years in Dallas, Texas, who are malnourished.

Tertiary Prevention

Tertiary prevention is the third level or therapeutic stage of prevention. The first two levels are primary and secondary. Tertiary prevention employs intervention strategies directed at assisting diseased and disabled people in a population to reduce the impact of their existing disabilities (Bates & Winder, 1984).

Tertiary prevention relies more heavily on medical care and rehabilitation than on health promotion and education. Much of patient education is tertiary prevention.

See **Primary Prevention** and **Secondary Prevention.**

Theory

A theory is the formation of principles and concepts used to predict and explain a phenomenon, such as human behavior. A theory is an integrated set of propositions intended to give deeper understanding of a philosophy and provide a basis for explaining certain happenings of life.

In the health education field, theories are developed to explain the processes underlying learning and offer program planners a framework or guide in selecting interventions needed to accomplish stated goals and objectives. Much of health education and promotion programs are planned and evaluated on the basis of proven theories (Powers & Knapp, 1990; Rosenstock et al., 1988; Ross & Mico, 1980).

See **Theory of Planned Behavior** and **Theory of Reasoned Action.**

Theory of Planned Behavior

The theory of planned behavior is an extension of the theory of reasoned action, and includes a person's attitudes toward a behavior. The use of this theory may have significant impact on the development of health programs, because it has been very successful in dealing with behaviors in which there is a conscious choice (Ajzen, 1991; Doll & Ajzen, 1992; Rodgers & Brawley, 1993; Wankel & Mummery, 1993).

See **Theory of Reasoned Action.**

Theory of Reasoned Action

The theory of reasoned action is a social-psychological model of voluntary behavior based on the assumption that intentions are the most immediate influence on behavior. The theory of reasoned action emphasizes the role of personal intention in determining whether or not a behavior will occur.

According to this theory, intentions are influenced by attitudes and subjective norms, or perceptions of social pressures. Attitudes are determined by beliefs about the consequences of behavior, and subjective norms are affected by the actions of significant others.

The theory was developed to explain behavior and provide a framework for studying attitudes toward behavior. It was extended to include the concept of perceived control as a third influence on intentions (Ajzen & Fishbein, 1980; Fishbein & Ajzen, 1975).

See **Behavioral Intention** and **Theory of Planned Behavior.**

Time Line

A time line is a working schedule developed and used in the planning and execution of a program or project to show the activities and the time they are expected to be accomplished during the course of the program. A time line usually delineates activities vertically on a page with a schedule of time (by day, month, or year depending on the period covered) presented horizontally.

See **Gannt Chart.**

Transtheoretical Model

The transtheoretical model was developed by two psychologists, James Prochaska and Carlo DiClemente, in 1984 to describe and explain stages that people go through during psychotherapy (Kaplan et al., 1993).

The transtheoretical model implies that as people pass through these stages of change (precontemplation, contemplation, decision, action, and maintenance) they may need different intervention approaches. Although not fully tested, the model has been useful in studying a variety of health behaviors, such as smoking. It has been applied in smoking cessation interventions and in alcohol treatment plans (DiClemente et al., 1991; DiClemente & Hughes, 1990). The model has also been applied to weight control (O'Connell & Velicer, 1988) and other health problems, including risk behavior related to AIDS.

See **Stages of Change.**

Type A Behavior

Type A behavior is a pattern of conduct and emotion characterized by competitiveness, aggression, hostility, and time urgency that has been suspected of being a risk factor for coronary heart disease. Hostility, or the cynical mistrust of other people, is seen as the "toxic core" of this behavior pattern and best predicts cardiovascular disease (CVD) and all-cause mortality.

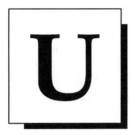

Unintentional Injury

Unintentional injuries are injuries or impairments such as those caused by motor vehicle collisions, fires, falls, drownings, and firearms. In the United States, injury is the leading cause of death and illness for people under the age of 45 years and the fourth leading cause of death for all ages (Dannenberg, Gielen, Beilenson, Wilson, & Joffe, 1993; Gielen, 1992; Martinez, 1990; "Setting the National Agenda," 1992).

Injury, now recognized as a public health problem needing attention, is a concern to public health professionals, policymakers, and the general public.

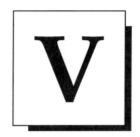

Validity

Validity is the degree to which a test or assessment measures what it is intended to measure. Using an acceptable (valid) instrument increases the chance of measuring what was intended (Vogt, 1993; Windsor et al., 1994).

Validity also refers to accuracy of a study or data collection instrument, and includes external as well as internal validity. It is the appropriateness or usefulness of specific inferences made from test scores, or the quality of data derived from the use of an instrument (questionnaire).

Forms of validity regularly used in health education evaluation are content validity, criterion-related validity, and construct validity.

See **Construct Validity, Content Validity, External Validity,** and **Internal Validity.**

Values

Values are highly esteemed cultural perspectives or beliefs shared and transmitted among people who hold a common history or identity. This term may not be appropriate for school-based health education, but may be meaningful to health education in other settings.

Values Clarification

Values clarification is a methodology or strategy dealing with techniques that help learners clarify, define, and defend their values about moral, ethical, social, and other relationships.

Values clarification emphasizes the processes that learners use to arrive at a value judgment and helps in the identification and clarification of their thinking regarding important issues, without indoctrinating or forcing them to take a position (Greenberg, 1975; Levinger & Toomey, 1982; Martin, 1982; Toohey & Valenzuela, 1983).

Voluntary Health Organization or Agency

A voluntary health organization is a nonprofit, nongovernmental association dedicated to providing health education and/or health services related to specific health concerns. Voluntary organizations are supported financially by contributions from individuals and agencies, and depend on volunteers to provide much of the work.

Examples: American Heart Association and American Cancer Society.

V

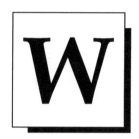

Weight Cycling

Weight cycling refers to the yo-yo diet syndrome of repeated weight losses and regains, which make it more and more difficult to lose body fat.

Wellness

Wellness is a dimension of health that goes beyond the absence of disease or infirmity and includes the integration of social, mental, emotional, spiritual, and physical aspects of health. The concept of wellness was first introduced in the United States in the 1970s as an expanding experience of purposeful and enjoyable living. Wellness refers to a positive stage, illness to a negative state (Butler, 1994; Green & Kreuter, 1991).

Wellness Center

Wellness centers are organized and operated mainly by health professionals, such as health education specialists, nurses, therapists, nutritionists, medical doctors with an interest in prevention, and health administrators to provide people with learning opportunities about health behavior and issues related to the health of the population. Learning opportunities may involve health education workshops, weight control clinics, exercise demonstrations, cooking demonstrations, nutrition classes, and stress management programs.

Work Plan

A work plan is a detailed description of the activities needed to reach stated objectives. Work plans must be written in a specific and detailed manner. They are tools that guide project implementation and should reflect the best projection of tasks, time lines, and evaluation points under the worst possible scenario.

Work Site Health Promotion

Work site health promotion is a program given at the place of employment or sponsored by employers to benefit employees, a high percent of whom may not otherwise participate in health promotion programs.

Health promotion at the work site covers a wide variety of activities, including exercise and fitness, stress management, smoking cessation, nutrition education, and cholesterol reduction. Specific programs targeting women include prenatal care, parenting, environmental influences affecting the outcome of pregnancy, Pap smears, and breast examinations and mammograms (Breslow, Fielding, Herman, & Wilbur, 1990; Fielding, 1990; Selleck, Sirles, & Newman, 1989).

Some work site health promotion efforts may require that employees engage in behaviors that protect their health, such as wearing hard hats, and not smoking or using alcohol on the job. The work site offers enormous potential for health promotion, and employees as well as employers share in the benefits. Some benefits from work site health promotion are better productivity, decreased absenteeism, improved employee health, improved employee morale, reduced work stress, healthy pregnancy and delivery outcomes, fewer babies with low birth weight, and enhanced sense of well-being (Chenoweth, 1991; Modeste, 1994).

Business and industry may employ health educators, nurse practitioners, physicians, physician assistants, and other health professionals to manage health promotion programs. Smaller businesses and corporations may cosponsor programs with larger ones.

W

PART TWO

Health and Professional Organizations

Health and Professional Organizations

Action on Smoking and Health (ASH)

This organization serves members and local groups. It focuses on publicizing the dangers of smoking through campaigns for a smoke-free public; promotes national No-Smoking Day; and liaises with health promotion organizations and private groups. ASH also disseminates information related to smoking and health and monitors scientific and trade publications. ASH publishes a biweekly Information Bulletin and a quarterly supporter newsletter.

Address for ASH: 109 Gloucester Place, London, W14 4DH, England.

Address for ASH Scottish branch: 8 Federick Street, Edinburgh, EH2 2HB, Scotland.

Agency for Health Care Policy and Research (AHCPR)

The Agency for Health Care Policy and Research (AHCPR) was created by Congress in 1989 within the Public Health Service. The agency is federally funded, focuses on health services research, and is devoted specifically to prevention.

The purpose of the agency is to enhance the quality of life of patient care services through improved knowledge that can be used in meeting the health care needs of society. AHCPR seeks to achieve its mission through several broad goals: the promotion of improvements in clinical practice and patient outcomes through more appropriate and effective health care services; the promotion of improvements in the financing, organization, and delivery of health care services; and the increase of access to high-quality care. The agency also sponsors individual and institutional National Research Service Awards, providing pre- and postdoctoral support for academics and for research concerning health services research methods and problems.

Agency for Toxic Substances and Disease Registry (ATSDR)

The Agency for Toxic Substances and Disease Registry (ATSDR) works to prevent adverse human health effects and diminished quality of life that can result from exposure to hazardous substances in the environment. ATSDR is administered by the director of the Centers for Disease Control and Prevention (CDC), but is a separate agency.

ATSDR evaluates data and information on the release of hazardous substances into the environment. It assesses any current or future effects on public health, develops health advisories, and identifies studies or actions needed to evaluate and mitigate or prevent adverse human health effects. ATSDR increases an understanding of the relationship between exposure to hazardous substances and adverse effects on human health through epidemiology, surveillance, and other studies on toxic substances and their effects.

ATSDR monitors people's exposure to hazardous substances through a registry of people exposed to hazardous substances, serious diseases, and illnesses. In addition, it provides health-related support to states, local agencies, and health care providers in public health care emergencies that involve exposure to hazardous substances, health consultations, and training.

The agency develops and makes available to physicians and other health care providers materials on the health effects of toxic substances and maintains a list of sites that are closed or restricted to the public because of contamination. Summaries of such materials may also be made available to the public.

ATSDR identifies gaps in knowledge, initiates research in toxicology and health effects where needed, and conducts or sponsors applied research on the human health effects of hazardous substances released into the environment from waste sites or other hazardous wastes.

Address for ATSDR: U.S. Department of Health and Human Services, Mail Stop SSOP, Washington, DC 20402-9328.

Alcohol, Drug Abuse, and
Mental Health Administration (ADAMHA)

The Alcohol, Drug Abuse, and Mental Health Administration (ADAMHA) leads national efforts to improve the scientific understanding of the causes, course, and effects of addictive mental disorders, and exerts national leadership to increase the nation's ability to prevent and treat these disorders.

The agency conducts biomedical as well as behavioral research on mental illness and substance abuse, then it translates the findings on cost-effective prevention and treatment programs through agencies such as the National Institute of Mental Health (NIMH), the National Institute on Alcohol Abuse and Alcoholism (NIAAA), and the National Institute on Drug Abuse (NIDA) (*see* **NIMH, NIAAA,** and **NIDA**).

Address for ADAMHA: U.S. Department of Health and Human Services, Mail Stop SSOP, Washington, DC 20402-9328.

American Alliance for Health, Physical Education,
Recreation and Dance (AAHPERD)

The American Alliance for Health, Physical Education, Recreation and Dance (AAHPERD) is made up of national associations:

1. Association for the Advancement of Health Education (AAHE)—dedicated to improving human health through health education (*see* **AAHE**)
2. American Association for Leisure and Recreation (AALR)—dedicated to enhancing the quality of life of the American people through the promotion of creative and meaningful leisure and recreation experiences
3. Association for Research, Administration, Professional Councils, and Societies (ARAPCS)—devoted to the pursuit and promotion of a healthy quality of life through services such as research, publication, and administration
4. National Association for Girls and Women in Sports (NAGWS)—fosters quality and equality in sports for girls and women, and serves those who coach, teach, and administer sports

127

5. National Association for Sport and Physical Education (NASPE)—devoted exclusively to improving the total sport and physical education experience in the United States

6. National Dance Association (NDA)—dedicated to promoting the development and implementation of philosophies and policies in all forms of dance and dance education

Address for AAHPERD and affiliates: 1900 Association Drive, Reston, Virginia 22091.

American College Health Association (ACHA)

The American College Health Association (ACHA) is a professional organization made up of individuals and institutions of higher education addressing health problems such as teenage pregnancy, sex education, AIDS issues, school health education and services, and other health-related issues in the academic community. The association promotes continuing education, research, and program development primarily for schools and educational institutions.

Address for ACHA: 2807 Central Street, Evanston, Illinois 60201.

American Public Health Association (APHA)

The American Public Health Association (APHA), founded in 1872, is the largest public health organization in the United States, and is committed to the protection and promotion of personal and environmental health and the prevention of disease.

APHA represents all disciplines and specialties of public health, and is active in policy development and special projects. The association plans annual conferences for the continuing professional development of its membership. The Public Health Promotion and Education and School Health Education and Services sections are especially relevant to the concerns of health educators.

APHA is responsible for the publication of the *American Journal of Public Health* and a newsletter, *The Nation's Health*.

Address for APHA: 1015 Fifteenth Street NW, Washington, DC 20005.

American School Health Association (ASHA)

The American School Health Association (ASHA) is the primary professional organization concerned with issues related to school-age children. School health services, healthful school environment, and comprehensive school health education are key areas of concern.

ASHA publishes the *American Journal of School Health.*

Address for ASHA: P.O. Box 708, Kent, Ohio 44240.

American Society for Healthcare
Education and Training (ASHET)

The American Society for Healthcare Education and Training (ASHET) is a membership organization representing a diversity of health care and educational organizations as well as health care individuals for the purpose of promoting awareness of the educational needs common to all health care personnel, continuation of professional development in management, and participation in national health issues.

ASHET is responsible for the journals *Hospital* and *Health Care Education.*

Address for ASHET: 840 North Lake Shore Drive, Chicago, Illinois 60611.

Association for the Advancement of Health Education (AAHE)

The Association for the Advancement of Health Education (AAHE) is one of six associations that make up the American Alliance for Health, Physical Education, Recreation and Dance (AAHPERD) (*see* **AAHPERD**). AAHE is a national professional membership organization representing thousands of health educators and health promotion specialists who work in schools, colleges and universities, medical care facilities, community and public health agencies, and business and industry.

AAHE members benefit from a subscription to the *Journal of Health Education* and *HE-XTRA,* a newsletter from the national AAHE office reporting on news and current events in health education. Members also benefit from conferences, conventions, and leadership opportunities.

Address for AAHE: 1900 Association Drive, Reston, Virginia 22091.

Association for Worksite Health Promotion (AWHP)

The Association for Worksite Health Promotion (AWHP) is a membership organization for health professionals committed to advancing work site health promotion throughout the world. Association members receive networking, education, resources, and recognition opportunities with their peers through annual international conferences dedicated exclusively to promoting work site health.

The association publishes a quarterly journal, *Worksite Health*, covering important issues and trends shaping the industry, and a bimonthly newsletter covering activities, news, promotions, conference highlights, and other member events.

Address for AWHP: c/o The Sherwood Group, 60 Revere Drive, Suite 500, Northbrook, Illinois 60062.

Association of State and Territorial Directors of Health Promotion and Public Health Education (ASTDHPPHE)

The Association of State and Territorial Directors of Health Promotion and Public Health Education (ASTDHPPHE) is made up of 65 directors of health education from the states and territories and the Indian Health Service of the United States. It is primarily concerned with developing standards of health education programming at the state level.

Address for ASTDHPPHE: Maine Bureau of Health, State House, Station 11, 151 Capitol Street, Augusta, Maine 04333-0011.

Black Health Research Foundation

This was formerly the Black Medical Research Foundation. It is a voluntary health agency devoted to reducing preventable causes of premature death among African Americans. The agency funds scientific research, promotes professional and community education, seeks to influence public policy on crucial health issues, and publishes the Black Health Column monthly, as well as a newsletter.

Address: 14 East 60th Street, Suite 307, New York, NY 10022.

Canadian Council on Smoking and Health (CCSH)

The Canadian Council on Smoking and Health (CCSH) helps to raise public awareness regarding the dangers of smoking, lobbies for smoke-free public areas, and disseminates information.

Address for CCSH: 1565 Carling Avenue, Suite 400, Ottawa, Ontario, Canada K1Z 8R1.

Canadian Public Health Association (CPHA)

The Canadian Public Health Association (CPHA) is a not-for-profit association for health professionals. CPHA supports health and social programs and represents public health in Canada with links to the international community.

The association provides members with an opportunity to speak out on broader public health issues, outside discipline boundaries. It aims at improving and maintaining personal and community health according to the public health principals of disease prevention, health promotion and protection, and healthy public policy.

The CPHA is responsible for several publications including the *Canadian Journal of Public Health*, a monthly professional journal, and a quarterly magazine titled *CPHA Health Digest*.

Address for CPHA: 1565 Carling Avenue, Suite 400, Ottawa, Ontario, Canada K1Z 8R1. (There are also provincial and territorial branch associations, and addresses may be obtained from the above address.)

Centers for Disease Control and Prevention (CDC)

The Centers for Disease Control and Prevention (CDC) were established as the Communicable Disease Center in 1946 in Atlanta, Georgia, and have directed efforts to prevent diseases such as malaria, polio, smallpox, toxic shock syndrome, Legionnaires disease, and more recently, acquired immunodeficiency syndrome (AIDS).

CDC is concerned with health education and promotion activities such as chronic disease prevention and control, tobacco prevention and control, and injury prevention and control. CDC is also involved in health surveillance and selected treatment activities that support prevention.

According to CDC advertising, the mission of the agency is to "promote health and quality of life by preventing and controlling disease, injury, and disability." Its vision is "Healthy People in a Healthy World Through Prevention." Its mission is accomplished through national and international leadership; applied epidemiologic, laboratory, and behavioral research; building the public health system through technical and financial assistance and training; setting standards and guidelines; and surveillance and data analysis. Research findings and surveillance data are published in the *Morbidity and Mortality Weekly Report*.

Address for CDC: 1600 Clifton Road NE, Atlanta, Georgia 30333.

Chinese Association on Smoking and Health (CASH)

This is a membership organization that conducts research and educational programs, compiles statistics on smoking and health, and publishes a quarterly newsletter.

Address: Building 12, District 1, Andingmenwai Anhuaxili, Beijing 100011, People's Republic of China.

Council on Education for Public Health (CEPH)

The Council on Education for Public Health (CEPH) is the national accreditation body for schools of public health and certain graduate public health education programs offered in education settings other than schools of public health.

CEPH aims at promoting quality in education for public health through a continuing process of self-evaluation by the schools and programs that seek accreditation; assuring the public that institutions offering accredited graduate instruction in public health meet standards essential to conduct such programs; and encouraging improvements in the quality of education for public health through periodic review, research, publication, and consultation. The council also establishes its own accreditation policies, procedures, and fees for consultation and accreditation.

Address for CEPH: 1015 Fifteenth Street NW, Washington, DC 20005.

Environmental Protection Agency (EPA)

The Environmental Protection Agency (EPA), created in 1970 as an independent agency of the U.S. government, is the primary federal agency charged with protecting the nation's land, air, and water systems.

EPA strives to formulate and implement actions to lead to a compatible balance between human activities and the ability of natural systems to support and nurture life. EPA is responsible for ensuring the enforcement of all federally mandated statutes concerning environmental health and environmental protection (Vincoli, 1993). In addition, EPA publishes a quarterly journal, *EPA Journal*.

Address for EPA Public Information Center: 401 M Street SW (PM-211B), Washington, DC 20460.

International Health Foundation (IHF)

The International Health Foundation is dedicated to advancing the health of humankind by defining human mental, physical, and social problems and contributing to their solutions. The IHF promotes research and education, conducts and publishes health-related studies, and publishes a quarterly Information Bulletin.

Address of IHF: 8 Avenue Don Bosco, B-1150, Brussels, Belgium.

International Planned Parenthood Federation (IPPF)

The IPPF is a nongovernmental, independent association that works to initiate and support family planning services, develop resources, and stimulate research. The IPPF provides several publications including a bimonthly medical bulletin.

Address for IPPF: Regent's College, Inner Circle, Regent's Park, London NW1 4NS, England.

International Society on Hypertension in Blacks (ISHIB)

The International Society on Hypertension in Blacks (ISHIB) is a nonprofit organization dedicated to improving the health and life expectancy of ethnic populations in the United States and around the world. The organization was founded in Atlanta, Georgia, in 1986 to respond to the problem of high blood pressure among Blacks and has since broadened its mission to include the total spectrum of ethnicity and disease.

ISHIB aims at stimulating research and clinical investigation; disseminating scientific findings to aid in the understanding of differences in hypertension among ethnic groups; promoting public awareness of the harmful effects of hypertension, especially among Blacks; educating the public on ways to prevent the complications of hypertension; and developing health-related programs to improve the quality of life of ethnic populations worldwide.

ISHIB contributes to world health through the Heart to Heart Program, offering life-saving surgery to children of families from developing countries where medical care is scarce and technology is still evolving. Children with life-threatening heart problems are brought to the United States for surgical care.

ISHIB sponsors yearly international conferences at different geographic locations, attracting people in the medical and health professions from throughout the world who want to learn firsthand the latest in research and clinical practice.

ISHIB publishes a newsletter, *ISHIB News,* and a quarterly journal, *Journal of Ethnicity and Disease.*

Address for ISHIB: 2045 Manchester Street NE, Atlanta, Georgia 30324-4110.

International Union for Health Promotion and Education (IUHPE)

The International Union for Health Promotion and Education (IUHPE) is an international professional organization committed to the development of health education around the world. Formerly the International Union for Health Education (IUHE), it now includes health promotion.

IUHPE has constituent, institutional, and individual memberships. It works closely with the World Health Organization (WHO) (*see* **WHO**) and the United Nations Educational, Scientific, and Cultural Organization (UNESCO) in a variety of forums.

IUHPE objectives are as follows:

1. To establish effective links between organizations and people in health education in several countries
2. To facilitate global exchange of information, experiences, and programs relating to health
3. To promote scientific research and improvement of professional preparation in health education

IUHPE publishes an international journal of health promotion and education, *Promotion and Education* (formerly *HYGIE*), and *NARO News.*

Address for North American Regional Office: P.O. Box 2305, Station D, Ottawa, Ontario, Canada K1P5KO.

National Commission for Health Education Credentialing (NCHEC)

The National Commission for Health Education Credentialing (NCHEC) is the official organization responsible for establishing, implementing, and maintaining a certification process for health education specialists through professional preparation and continuing education. Its mission is to improve the quality of health education practice and to ensure continual updating of skills and knowledge.

This organization was established in 1988 and became incorporated as a nonprofit, tax-exempt organization with an elected board of directors. In the early stages of the organization, experienced health educators were permitted to apply for charter certification, but as of 1990, individuals become certified by passing an examination. Recertification is made available every 5 years based on continuing education criteria.

Address for NCHEC: 475 Riverside Drive, Suite 740, New York, New York 10115.

National Council for the Education of Health Professionals in Health Promotion (NCEHPHP)

The National Council for the Education of Health Professionals in Health Promotion (NCEHPHP) works with institutions that train allied health professionals, as well as public health and primary care professionals, preparing them to incorporate health promotion and disease prevention in their curriculum, certification, and continuing education activities. Its mission is to ensure that all health professionals are adequately prepared to make health promotion and disease prevention components of their practice.

Address for NCEHPHP: American College of Preventive Medicine, 1015 Fifteenth Street NW, Suite 403, Washington, DC 20005.

National Institute of Mental Health (NIMH)

The National Institute of Mental Health (NIMH) is the largest scientific institute in the world with a primary focus on mental disorders. The institute directs federal efforts to promote mental health, prevent and treat brain disorders and mental illness, and rehabilitate those who suffer from mental conditions.

NIMH conducts and supports research on the biological, psychological, behavioral, clinical, and epidemiological aspects of mental health and on disorders of the brain and mind. In addition, it funds the training of researchers; provides professional assistance to the states and community organizations responsible for mental health programs; and disseminates research findings to health care professionals, the media, and the public.

Address for NIMH: U.S. Department of Health and Human Services, Mail Stop SSOP, Washington, DC 20402-9328.

National Institute on Alcohol Abuse and Alcoholism (NIAAA)

The National Institute on Alcohol Abuse and Alcoholism (NIAAA) leads the federal government's efforts to reduce the enormous health, social, and economic consequences of alcohol abuse and alcoholism. NIAAA operates a research program encompassing a wide range of research in the biomedical and behavioral sciences.

NIAAA supports intramural research facilities, promotes a variety of research efforts, and fosters the development of effective treatment and prevention through the circulation of research findings to health care providers. The institute has also expanded research on public policy issues such as alcohol taxation, alcohol consumption, warning labels, and drinking and driving laws to provide a scientific basis for the development and assessment of public policy.

Address for NIAAA: U.S. Department of Health and Human Services, Mail Stop SSOP, Washington, DC 20402-9328.

National Institute on Drug Abuse (NIDA)

The National Institute on Drug Abuse (NIDA) is the leading federal agency for research on the incidence and prevalence of drug abuse, its causes and consequences, and improved methods of prevention and treatment of drug abuse, with the intention of increasing knowledge and solving problems associated with drug abuse.

NIDA supports research on effective prevention and treatment of drug abuse and on the role of drug abuse as a factor in the spread of AIDS. Research findings are usually presented in NIDA research monographs, available from the U.S. Department of Health and Human Services.

Address for NIDA: U.S. Department of Health and Human Services, National Institute on Drug Abuse, 5600 Fishers Lane, Rockville, MD 20857.

Society for Public Health Education (SOPHE)

The Society for Public Health Education (SOPHE) is a national professional service organization formed in 1950 to promote, encourage, and contribute to the health of all people by stimulating research, developing criteria for professional preparation, elevating performance standards for the practice of health education, promoting networking among health education professionals, and advocating policy and legislation affecting health education and health promotion.

SOPHE is the only professional organization devoted exclusively to public health education and health promotion. The organization is responsible for the *Health Education Quarterly* journal, one of the most widely cited journals in the *Social Sciences Index,* and a quarterly newsletter, *News and Views.*

SOPHE sponsors annual and midyear scientific conferences, and offers continuing education contact hours at conferences and workshops for Certified Health Education Specialists (CHESs) (*see* **CHES**). SOPHE also works with advisory boards and coalitions at the national, state, and local levels to influence health promotion practice and policy decisions. It serves to stimulate peer exchange through its annual membership directory and supports ethical health education research by promoting the SOPHE Code of Ethics (*see* **Ethics**).

SOPHE recognizes professional excellence and leadership through Distinguished Fellow, Student Paper, and Program Excellence Awards. The society has many chapters in many states.

Address for SOPHE: 2001 Addison Street, Suite 220, Berkeley, California 94704.

United Nations International Children's Emergency Fund (UNICEF)

The United Nations International Children's Emergency Fund (UNICEF), or United Nations Children's Fund, was established after World War II to assist children in wartorn Europe, mainly through the distribution of powdered milk from the United States. As conditions improved, attention expanded from Europe to the world's needy children. UNICEF instituted programs to control yaws, tuberculosis, and leprosy and to provide clean drinking water and education to improve the health of children globally.

UNICEF was a cosponsor of the Alma Ata conference in 1978 on primary health care (*see* **Alma Ata Declaration**). Funding is through contributions, sale of greeting cards, monies from government and nongovernmental organizations, and other sources (Basch, 1990).

Address for UNICEF: UNICEF House, 3 United Nations Plaza, New York, New York 10017.

Worksite Health Promotion Alliance (WHPA)

The Worksite Health Promotion Alliance (WHPA), founded by Bill Whitmer and others, is a coalition of organizations and associations that represent small and large businesses interested in work site health promotion programs. WHPA is endorsed by professional groups and individuals with expertise in work site health promotion.

WHPA is administered by a board of directors made up of corporate executives, physicians, economists, academics, scientists, providers, and executive directors of large national organizations and associations.

Address for WHPA: 2040 Valleydale Road, Suite 202, Birmingham, Alabama 35244. Telephone: (205) 988-4441.

World Health Organization (WHO)

The World Health Organization (WHO) is an agency of the United Nations that serves as the premier organization in the field of health worldwide. It was established shortly after World War II on April 7, 1948, a day annually commemorated as World Health Day. Intended to assist people in attaining the best possible health, WHO is financed by dues from member countries, voluntary funds, and contributions from several sources.

Headquartered in Geneva, with six regional headquarters (Europe, Eastern Mediterranean, Africa, Southeast Asia, Western Pacific, and the Americas) and collaborating centers and offices in many countries, WHO provides services to governments and central technical services such as information on health aspects of travel and commerce, international standardization of vaccines and pharmaceuticals, and literature disseminating knowledge on world health problems. WHO is committed to the immunization of the world's children.

WHO has a fellowship program administered through regional offices where people can receive short study tours abroad in public health administration, nursing, environmental health, maternal and child health, and other disciplines. Services to governments are usually at the request of member countries for specific projects, and for training health personnel. WHO also assists governments in reviewing and evaluating health needs and resources.

Address for WHO: Regional Office, 525 Twenty-third Street NW, Washington, DC 20037.

Most of the organizations listed in this section have their counterpart associations in several countries. There are also other health agencies, both national and international, not mentioned.

References

Ajzen, I. (1991). The theory of planned behavior. *Organizational Behavior and Human Decision Processes, 50*(2), 179-211.

Ajzen, I., & Fishbein, M. (1980). *Understanding attitudes and predicting social behavior.* Englewood Cliffs, NJ: Prentice Hall.

Allensworth, D. D., & Kolbe, L. J. (1987). The comprehensive school health program: Exploring an expanded concept. *Journal of School Health, 57,* 409-411.

Alonzo, A. A. (1984). An illness behavior paradigm: A conceptual exploration of a situational-adaptation perspective. *Social Science and Medicine, 19*(5), 499-510.

Anderson, C. L., & Creswell, W. H. (1980). *School health practice.* St. Louis, MO: C. V. Mosby.

Anderson, L. A., DeVellis, R. F., Sharpe, P. A., & Marcoux, B. (1994). Multidimensional health locus of control scales: Do they measure expectancies about control or desires for control? *Health Education Research, 9*(1), 145-151.

Anderson, S. V., & Bauwens, E. E. (1981). *Chronic health problems: Concepts and applications.* St. Louis, MO: C. V. Mosby.

Antonovsky, A. (1980). *Health, stress, and coping.* San Francisco: Jossey-Bass.

Aronson, E. (1992). The return of the repressed: Dissonance theory makes a comeback. *Psychological Inquiry, 3*(4), 303-311.

Association for the Advancement of Health Education. (1994). Code of ethics for health educators. *Journal of Health Education, 25*(4), 197-200.

Backett, K., Davison, C., & Mullen, K. (1994). Lay evaluation of health and healthy lifestyles: Evidence from three studies. *British Journal of General Practice, 44*(383), 277-280.

Bandura, A. (1971). *Psychological modeling.* Chicago: Atherton.

Bandura, A. (1977). *Social learning theory.* Englewood Cliffs, NJ: Prentice Hall.

Bandura, A. (1982). Self-efficacy mechanisms in human agency. *American Psychologist, 37,* 122-147.

Banwell, J. G. (1990). Worldwide impact of oral rehydration therapy. *Clinical Therapy, 12*(Suppl. A), 29-36.

Baranowski, T. (1989-1990). Reciprocal determinism at the stages of behavior change: An integrational community, personal, and behavioral perspectives. *International Quarterly of Community Health Education, 10*(4), 297-327.

Barnes, S., Fors, S., & Becker, W. (1980). Ethical issues in health education. *Health Education, 11*(2), 7-9.

Basch, C. E., Eveland, J. D., & Portnoy, B. (1986). Diffusion systems for education and learning about health. *Family and Community Health, 9*(2), 1-26.

Basch, P. F. (1990). *Textbook of international health.* New York: Oxford University Press.

Bates, I., & Winder, A. (1984). *Introduction to health education.* Mountain View, CA: Mayfield.

Bauer, R. A. (Ed.). (1966). *Social indicators.* Cambridge: MIT Press.

Beach, L. R., & Wise, J. A. (1980). Decision emergence: A Lewinian perspective. *Acta Psychologica, 45*(1-3), 343-356.

Becker, M. H. (1974). *The Health Belief Model and personal health behavior.* Thorofare, NJ: Charles B. Slack.

Bedworth, A. E., & Bedworth, D. A. (1992). *The profession and practice of health education.* Dubuque, IA: Brown & Benchmark.

Bellock, N. B., & Breslow, L. (1972). Relationship of physical health status and health practice. *Preventive Medicine, 1,* 409-421.

Belzer, E. G., & McIntyre, L. (1994). A model for coordinating school health promotion programs. *Journal of School Health, 64*(5), 196-200.

Benenson, A. (1990). *Control of communicable diseases in man.* Washington, DC: American Public Health Association.

Bloom, B. S. (Ed.). (1956). *Taxonomy of educational objectives. Handbook 1: Cognitive domain.* New York: David MacKay.

Bloomquist, K. B. (1986). Modeling and health behavior: Strategies for prevention in schools. *Health Education, 17*(3), 8-11.

Bossert, T. J., & Parker, D. A. (1984). The political and administrative context of primary health care in the third world. *Social Science and Medicine, 18,* 693-702.

Bracht, N. (Ed.). (1990). *Health promotion at the community level.* Newbury Park, CA: Sage.

Brandon, P. (1993). School health services—A dimension of health care reform. *Oregon Nurse, 58*(2), 7-8.

Breckon, D. J., Harvey, J. R., & Lancaster, R. B. (1989). *Community health education.* Rockville, MD: Aspen.

Breckon, D. J., Harvey, J. R., & Lancaster, R. B. (1994). *Community health education: Settings, roles and skills for the 21st century* (3rd ed.). Rockville, MD: Aspen.

Breslow, L., Fielding, J., Herman, A. A., & Wilbur, C. S. (1990). Worksite health promotion: Its evolution and the Johnson & Johnson experience. *Preventive Medicine, 19*(1), 13-21.

Brindis, C. (1993). Health policy reform and comprehensive school health education: The need for an effective partnership. *Journal of School Health, 63*(1), 33-37.

Bryant, C., & Gulitz, E. (1993). Focus group discussions: An application to teaching. *Journal of Health Education, 24*(3), 188-189.

Bunting, C. E. (1981). The development and validation of the education attitudes inventory. *Educational and Psychological Measurement, 41*(2), 559-565.

Bunton, R., & Macdonald, G. (1992). *Health promotion: Disciplines and diversity.* New York: Routledge, Chapman, & Hall.

Butler, J. T. (1994). *Principles of health promotion and education.* Englewood, CO: Morton.

Carey, V., Chapman, S., & Gaffney, D. (1994). Children's lives and garden aesthetics? A case study in public health advocacy. *Australian Journal of Public Health, 18*(1), 25-32.

Carkenord, D. M., & Bullington, J. (1993). Bringing cognitive dissonance to the classroom. *Teaching of Psychology, 20*(1), 41-43.

Carlaw, R. (1982). *Perspectives on community health education: A series of case studies.* Oakland, CA: Third Party Publishing.

Carlaw, R. W., & Ward, W. B. (1988). *Primary health care: The African experience.* Oakland, CA: Third Party Publishing.

Cartwright, S. (1993). Cooperative learning can occur in any kind of program. *Young Children, 48*(2), 12-14.

Casteel, H. B., & Fiedorek, S. C. (1990). Oral rehydration therapy. *Pediatric Clinic North America, 37*(2), 295-311.

Chenoweth, D. H. (1991). *Planning health promotion at the worksite* (2nd ed.). Dubuque, IA: Brown & Benchmark.

Cleary, H. P., Kichen, J. M., & Ensor, P. G. (1985). *Advancing health through education: A case study approach.* Mountain View, CA: Mayfield.

Cleary, M. J. (1993a). Credentialing and vendorship: Are we ready? *Journal of Health Education, 24*(5), 285-287.

Cleary, M. J. (1993b). Using portfolios to assess student performance in school health education. *Journal of School Health, 63*(9), 377-381.

Cobb, S. (1976). Social support as a moderator of life stress. *Psychosomatic Medicine, 38,* 300-313.

Cook, T. D., & Campbell, D. T. (1979). *Quasi-experimentation: Design and analysis for field settings.* Boston: Houghton Mifflin.

Cook, T. D., & Reichardt, C. S. (Eds.). (1979). *Qualitative and quantitative methods in evaluation research.* Beverly Hills, CA: Sage.

Cooper, J. (1992). Dissonance and the return of the self-concept. *Psychological Inquiry, 3*(4), 320-323.

Cornacchia, H. J., & Barrett, S. (1980). *Consumer health: A guide to intelligent decisions.* St. Louis, MO: C. V. Mosby.

Cornacchia, H. J., Olsen, H. K., & Nickerson, C. J. (1991). *Health in elementary schools.* St. Louis, MO: Mosby Year Book.

Cowley, S. (1994). Collaboration in health care: The education link. *Health Visit, 67*(1), 13-15.

Creswell, J. W. (1994). *Research design: Qualitative and quantitative approaches.* Thousand Oaks, CA: Sage.

Curry, S., Marlatt, G. A., & Gordon, J. R. (1987). Abstinence violation effect: Validation of an attributional construct with smoking cessation. *Journal of Consulting and Clinical Psychology, 55*(2), 145-149.

Dannenberg, A. L., Gielen, A. C., Beilenson, P. L., Wilson, M. H., & Joffe, A. (1993). Bicycle helmet laws and educational campaigns: An evaluation of strategies to increase children's helmet use. *American Journal of Public Health, 83*(5), 667-674.

Davis, R. G. (1985, Winter). Congress and the emergence of public health policy. *HCM Review,* pp. 61-72.

Delbecq, A. L. (1974). Contextual variables affecting decision making in program planning. *Decision Sciences, 5*(4), 726-742.

de Lissovoy, G., Rice, T., Gabel, J., & Gelzer, H. (1987). Preferred provider organizations one year later. *Inquiry, 24,* 127-139.

Deniston, O., & Rosenstock, I. (1968). Evaluation of program effectiveness. *Public Health Reports, 83*(4), 323-335.

DesCamp, K. D., & Thomas, C. C. (1993). Buffering nursing stress through play at work. *Western Journal of Nursing Research, 15*(5), 619-627.

Dever, G. E. (1976). An epidemiological model for health policy analysis. *Social Indicators Research, 2,* 453-466.

Diamond, G. A. (1992). Field theory and rational choice: A Lewinian approach to modeling motivation. *Journal of Social Issues, 48*(2), 79-94.

DiClemente, C. C., & Hughes, S. O. (1990). Stages of change profiles in outpatient alcoholism treatment. *Journal of Substance Abuse, 2,* 217-237.

DiClemente, C. C., Prochaska, J. O., Fairhurst, S. K., Velicer, W. F., Valasquez, M. M., & Rossi, J. S. (1991). The process of smoking cessation: An analysis of precontemplation, contemplation, and preparation stages of change. *Journal of Consulting and Clinical Psychology, 59,* 292-304.

Doll, J., & Ajzen, I. (1992). Accessibility and stability of predictors in the theory of planned behavior. *Journal of Personality and Social Psychology, 63*(5), 754-765.

Dorken, H. (1989). Hospital practice as gatekeeper to continuity of care: CHAMPUS mental health services: 1980-1987. *Professional Psychology Research and Practice, 20*(6), 419-420.

Emlet, C. A., & Hall, A. M. (1991). Integrating the community into geriatric case management: Public health interventions. *Gerontologist, 31*(4), 556-560.

Fenlason, K. J., & Beehr, T. A. (1994). Social support and occupational stress: Effects of talking to others. *Journal of Organizational Behavior, 15,* 157-175.

Festinger, L. (1957). *A theory of cognitive dissonance.* Stanford, CA: Stanford University Press.

Fielding, J. E. (1990). Worksite health promotion survey: Smoking control activities. *Preventive Medicine, 19*(4), 402-413.

Fink, A., & Kosecoff, J. (1979). *How to write and evaluate a report. How to evaluate health programs.* Washington, DC: Capitol Publications.

Fish, L. S., & Piercy, F. P. (1987). The theory and practice of structural and strategic family therapies: A Delphi study. *Journal of Marital and Family Therapy, 13*(20), 113-125.

Fishbein, M., & Ajzen, I. (1975). *Belief, attitude, intention and behavior.* Reading, MA: Addison-Wesley.

Foreyt, J. P., Goodrick, G. K., Reeves, R. S., & Raynaud, A. S. (1993). Response of free-living adults to behavioral treatment of obesity: Attrition and compliance to exercise. *Behavior Therapy, 24*(4), 659-669.

Fox, J. P., Hall, C. E., & Elveback, L. R. (1970). *Epidemiology: Man and disease.* New York: Macmillan.

Frankel, B. G., & Nuttall, S. (1984). Illness behavior: An exploration of determinants. *Social Science and Medicine, 19*(2), 147-155.

Friedman, G. D. (1980). *Primer of epidemiology.* New York: McGraw-Hill.

Furst, E. J. (1981). Bloom's taxonomy of educational objectives for the cognitive domain: Philosophical and educational issues. *Review of Educational Research, 51*(4), 441-453.

Gardner, W. I., & Cole, C. L. (1987). Managing aggressive behavior: A behavioral diagnostic approach. *Psychiatric Aspects of Mental Retardation Reviews, 6*(5), 21-25.

Gielen, A. C. (1992). Health education and injury control: Integrating approaches. *Health Education Quarterly, 19*(2), 1203-1218.

Gilmore, G. D., Campbell, M. D., & Becker, B. L. (1989). *Needs assessment strategies for health education and health promotion.* Indianapolis, IN: Benchmark.

Girvan, J. T., Hamburg, M. V., & Miner, K. R. (1993). Credentialing the health education profession. *Journal of Health Education, 24*(5), 260.

Glantz, K., Lewis, F. M., & Rimer, B. K. (1990). *Health behavior and health education: Theory, research and practice.* San Francisco: Jossey-Bass.

Glantz, L. H., Mariner, W. K., & Annas, G. J. (1992). Risky business: Setting public health policy for HIV-infected health care professionals. *Milbank Quarterly, 70*(1), 43-47.

Goodman, S. H., Cooley, E., Sewell, D. R., & Leavitt, N. (1994). Locus of control and self-esteem in depressed, low-income African American women. *Community Mental Health Journal, 30*(3), 259-269.

Graeff, J. A., Elder, T. P., & Mills-Booth, E. (1993). *Communication for health and behavior change.* San Francisco: Jossey-Bass.

Green, L. W., & Kreuter, M. W. (1991). *Health promotion planning: An educational and environmental approach.* Mountain View, CA: Mayfield.

Green, L. W., Kreuter, M. W., Deeds, S. G., & Partridge, K. B. (1980). *Health education planning: A diagnostic approach.* Mountain View, CA: Mayfield.

Greenberg, J. S. (1975). Behavior modification and values clarification and their research implications. *Journal of School Health, 45*(2), 91-95.

Greenberg, J. S. (1992). *Health education.* Dubuque, IA: William C. Brown.

Greenberg, J. S., & Gold, R. (1992). *The health education ethics book.* Dubuque, IA: Brown & Benchmark.

Grover, S. A., Gray, D. K., Joseph, L., Abrahamowicz, M., & Coupal, L. (1994). Life expectancy following dietary modification or smoking cessation. Estimating the benefits of a prudent lifestyle. *Archives of Internal Medicine, 154*(15), 1697-1704.

Grunbaum, J. A., Basen-Engquist, K. (1993). Comparison of health risk behaviors between students in a regular high school and students in an alternative high school. *Journal of School Health, 63*(10), 421-425.

Hall, S. M., Munoz, R. F., & Reus, V. I. (1994). Cognitive-behavioral intervention increases abstinence rates for depressive-history smokers. *Journal of Consulting and Clinical Psychology, 62*(1), 141-146.

Hamburg, M. V. (1993). Perspectives on teaching comprehensive school health. *Preventive Medicine, 22*(4), 533-543.

Handler, A., Schieve, L. A., Ippoliti, P., Gordon, A. K., & Turnock, B. J. (1994). Building bridges between schools of public health and public health practice. *American Journal of Public Health, 84*(7), 1077-1080.

Hanlon, J. J., & Pickett, G. E. (1984). *Public health administration and practice.* St. Louis, MO: C. V. Mosby.

Health Education Quarterly. (1994, Summer). *21*(2,3).

Herman, C. P., & Polivy, J. (1980). Restrained eating. In A. J. Stunkard (Ed.), *Obesity* (pp. 208-225). Philadelphia: W. B. Saunders.

Himsl, R., & Lambert, E. (1993). Signs of learning in the affective domain. *Alberta Journal of Educational Research, 39*(2), 257-273.

Hochbaum, G. (1980). Ethical dilemmas in health education. *Health Education, 11*(2), 4-6.

Holyoak, K. J., Koh, K., & Nisbett, R. E. (1989). A theory of conditioning: Inductive learning within rule-based default hierarchies. *Psychological Review, 96*(2), 315-340.

Howze, E. H., & Redman, L. J. (1992). The uses of theory in health advocacy: Policies and programs. *Health Education Quarterly, 19*(3), 369-383.

Hunt, M. K., Lefebvre, R. C., Hixson, M. L., Banspach, S. W., Assaf, A. R., & Carleton, R. A. (1990). Pawtucket heart health program point-of-purchase nutrition education program in supermarkets. *American Journal of Public Health, 80*(6), 730-732.

Israel, B. A., Checkoway, B., Schulz, A., & Zimmerman, M. (1994). Health education and community empowerment: Conceptualizing and measuring perceptions of individual, organizational, and community control. *Health Education Quarterly, 21*(2), 149-170.

Jackson, S. A. (1994). Comprehensive school health education programs: Innovative practices and issues in standard setting. *Journal of School Health, 64*(3), 177.

James, L. D., Thorn, B. E., & Williams, D. A. (1993). Goal specification in cognitive-behavioral therapy for chronic headache pain. *Behavior Therapy, 24*(2), 305-320.

Kaplan, G. M. (1991). The use of biofeedback in the treatment of chronic facial tics: A case study. *Medical Psychotherapy, an International Journal, 4*, 71-76.

Kaplan, M. (1988). Health related quality of life in cardiovascular disease. *Journal of Consulting and Clinical Psychology, 56*, 382-392.

Kaplan, R. M., Sallis, J. F., Jr., & Patterson, T. L. (1993). *Health and human behavior.* San Francisco: McGraw-Hill.

Kaufmann, P. (1973). Field theory and psychoanalysis: Introduction to Kurt Lewin. *Confrontations Psychiatriques, 6*(11), 223-249.

Keys, A., Brozek, J., Henschel, A., Michelson, O., & Taylor, H. L. (1950). *The biology of human starvation* (Vols. 1 & 2). Minneapolis: University of Minnesota Press.

Kickbusch, I. (1989). Self-care in health promotion. *Social Science and Medicine, 29*(2), 125-130.

Kish, L. (1987). *Statistical design for research.* New York: John Wiley.

Klein, D. (1968). *Community dynamic and mental health.* New York: John Wiley.

Knutsen, S. F. (1994). Lifestyle and the use of health services. *American Journal of Clinical Nutrition, 59*(Suppl. 5), 1171s-1175s.

Kotler, P. (1975). *Marketing for non-profit organizations.* Englewood Cliffs, NJ: Prentice Hall.

Kotler, P. (1982). *Marketing for nonprofit organizations.* Englewood Cliffs, NJ: Prentice Hall.

Kramer, M. S. (1988). *Clinical epidemiology and biostatistics.* New York: Springer-Verlag.

Kress, J. R., & Singer, J. (1975). *HMO handbook.* Rockville, MD: Aspens Systems.

Kreuger, R. (1989). *Focus groups: A practical guide for applied research.* Thousand Oaks, CA: Sage.

Kunstel, F. (1978). Assessing community needs: Implications for curriculum and staff development in health education. *Journal of School Health, 48*, 220-224.

Laberge, B., Gauthier, J. G., Cote, G., Plamondon, J., & Cormier, H. J. (1993). Cognitive behavioral therapy of panic disorder with secondary major depression: A preliminary investigation. *Journal of Consulting and Clinical Psychology, 61*(6), 1028-1037.

Labonte, R. (1989). Community empowerment: The need for political analysis. *Canadian Journal of Public Health, 80*, 87-88.

Labonte, R. (1994). Health promotion and empowerment: Reflections on professional practice. *Health Education Quarterly, 21*(2), 253-268.

Langwell, K. M. (1990). Structure and performance of health maintenance organizations: A review. *Health Care Financial Review, 12*(1), 71-80.

Lasater, T. M., Sennett, L. L., Lefebvre, R. C., DeHart, K. L., Peterson, G., & Carleton, R. A. (1991). Community-based approach to weight loss: The Pawtucket "weigh-in." *Addictive Behavior, 16*(3-4), 175-181.

Laser, E. D. (1985). An Adlerian approach to weight control, incorporating behavior modification techniques. *Individual Psychology Journal of Adlerian Theory, Research and Practice, 41*(2), 127-135.

Lee, P. R., & Estes, C. (1990). *The nation's health.* Boston: Jones & Bartlett.

Lee, S. S. (1982). Acquisition of inductive biconditional reasoning skills: Training of simultaneous and sequential processing. *Contemporary Educational Psychology, 7*(4), 371-383.

Lefebvre, R. C., Lasatar, T. M., Carleton, R. A., & Peterson, G. (1987). Theory and delivery of health programming in the community: The Pawtucket heart health program. *Preventive Medicine, 16*(1), 80-95.

Lester, D. (1990). Maslow's hierarchy of needs and personality. *Personality and Individual Differences, 11*(11), 1187-1188.

Lester, D., Hvezda, J., Sullivan, S., & Plourde, R. (1983). Maslow's hierarchy of needs and psychological health. *Journal of General Psychology, 109*(1), 83-85.

Levinger, L., & Toomey, B. (1982). A values-clarification group with adolescents. *Social Work in Health Care, 8*(1), 95-98.

Lilienfeld, A. M., & Lilienfeld, D. E. (1980). *Foundations of epidemiology.* New York: Oxford University Press.

Lipkin, J. O. (1980). Understanding illness behavior and its importance in the practice of medicine. *Behavioral Medicine Update, 2*, 15-18.

Livingood, W. C., Woodhouse, L. D., Godin, S., Eickmeier, J., Cosgrove, W., & Howard, M. (1993). Credentialing and competition for social jurisdiction. *Journal of Health Education, 24*(5), 282-284.

Lowis, A. (1992). Moving to a community based curriculum. *Occupational Health London, 44*(12), 368.

Lupton, D. (1994). Toward the development of critical health communication praxis. *Health Communication, 6*(1), 55-67.

Mail, P. D. (1993). A national profile of health educators: Preliminary data from the first cohorts of CHES. *Journal of Health Education, 24*(5), 269-277.

Marlatt, G. A., & Gordon, J. R. (1985). *Relapse prevention: Maintenance strategies in the treatment of addictive behaviors.* New York: Guilford.

Martin, G., & Pear, J. (1992). *Behavior modification.* Englewood Cliffs, NJ: Prentice Hall.

Martin, R. P. (1982). Values clarification: The state of the art for the 1980s—An interview with Sidney Simon and Howard Kirschenbaum. *Counseling and Values, 26*(4), 220-227.

Martinez, R. (1990). Injury control: A primer for physicians. *Annals of Emergency Medicine, 19*(1), 72-77.

Matarazzo, J. D., Weiss, S. M., Herd, J. A., Miller, M. E., & Weiss, S. M. (1984). *Behavioral health: A handbook of health enhancement and disease prevention.* New York: John Wiley.

Mayou, R. (1984). Sick role, illness behavior and coping. *British Journal of Psychiatry, 144,* 320-322.

McKenzie, J. F., & Jurs, J. L. (1993). *Planning, implementing, and evaluating health programs.* New York: Macmillan.

McMahon, R. C., Schram, L. L., & Davidson, R. S. (1993). Negative life events, social support, and depression in three personality types. *Journal of Personality Disorders, 7*(3), 241-254.

McMaster, C., & Lee, C. (1991). Cognitive dissonance in tobacco smokers. *Addictive Behaviors, 16*(5), 349-353.

Mico, P. R. (1978). An introduction to policy for health educators. *Health Education Monographs* (Supplement), *6,* 7-24.

Mielke, D. R. (1994). Health services for the health educator. *Journal of Health Education, 25*(4), 219-222.

Modeste, N. N. (1994). Worksite health promotion for women. *Promotion and Education, 1*(1), 29-33.

Moorhead, R. G. (1992). Who do people talk to about healthy lifestyles? A South Australian survey. *Family Practice, 9*(4), 472-475.

National Task Force on the Preparation and Practice of Health. (1985). *A framework for the development of competency-based curricula.* Berkeley, CA: Society for Public Health Education.

Nyswander, D. (1967). The open society: Its implications for health educators. *Health Education Monographs, 22*(4), 3-15.

O'Connell, D. O., & Velicer, W. F. (1988). A decisional balance measure and the stages of change model for weight loss. *International Journal of the Addictions, 23,* 729-750.

Okebukola, P. A. (1985). The relative effectiveness of cooperative learning interaction techniques in strengthening students' performance in science classes. *Science Education, 69*(4), 501-509.

Ornish, D., Brown, S. E., Scherwitz, L. W., et al. (1990). Can lifestyle changes reverse heart disease? The lifestyle heart trial. *Lancet, 336*(8708), 129-133.

Ovrebo, B., Ryan, M., Jackson, K., & Hutchinson, K. (1994). The homeless prenatal program: A model for empowering homeless pregnant women. *Health Education Quarterly, 21*(2), 187-198.

Owen, N. (1989). Behavioral intervention studies and behavioral epidemiology research to improve smoking-cessation strategies. *Health Education Research, 4*(1), 145-153.

Oyster, C. K., Hanten, W. P., & Llorens, L. A. (1987). *Introduction to research: A guide for the health science professional.* Philadelphia: J. B. Lippincott.

Patterson, S. M., & Vitello, E. M. (1993). Ethics in health education: The need to include a model course in professional preparation programs. *Journal of Health Education, 24*(4), 239-243.

Porritt, D. (1979). Social support in crisis: Quantity or quality? *Social Science and Medicine, 13A,* 715-721.

Portnoy, B., Anderson, D. M., & Eriksen, M. P. (1989). Application of diffusion theory to health promotion research. *Family and Community Health, 12*(3), 63-71.

Powers, B. A., & Knapp, T. (1990). *A dictionary of nursing theory and research.* Newbury Park, CA: Sage.

Pratkanis, A. R., Breckler, S. J., & Greenwald, A. G. (1989). *Attitude structure and function.* Hillsdale, NJ: Lawrence Erlbaum.

Quality of life as a new public health measure—Behavioral risk factor surveillance systems, 1993. (1994). *Morbidity and Mortality Weekly Report, 43,* 375-380.

Rajecki, B. W. (1990). *Attitudes.* Sutherland, MA: Sinauer.

Redican, K. J., Olsen, L. K., & Baffi, C. R. (1986). *Organization of school health programs.* New York: Macmillan.

Reid, W. M., Peace, J., & Taylor, R. G. (1990). The Delphi technique as an aid to organization development activities. *Organization Development Journal, 8*(3), 37-42.

Reinke, W. A. (1988). *Health planning for effective management.* New York: Oxford University Press.

Revenson, T. A., & Majerovitz, S. D. (1991). The effects of chronic illness on the spouse: Social resources as stress buffers. *Arthritis Care and Research, 4*(2), 63-72.

Ritchie, J. E. (1994). Education for primary health care: Accommodating the new realities. *World Health Forum, 15*(2), 147-149.

Rodin, J. (1980). The externality theory today. In A. J. Stunkard (Ed.), *Obesity* (pp. 226-239). Philadelphia: W. B. Saunders.

Rodgers, W. M., & Brawley, L. R. (1993). Using both self-efficacy theory and the theory of planned behavior to discriminate adherers and dropouts from structured programs. *Journal of Applied Sport Psychology, 5*(2), 195-206.

Rogers, E. M. (1983). *Diffusion of innovations* (3rd ed.). New York: Free Press.

Roper, W. L. (1993). Health communication takes on new dimensions at CDC. *Public Health Reports, 108*(2), 179.

Rose, S. M. (1986). Community organization: A survival strategy for community-based, empowerment-oriented programs. *Journal of Sociology and Social Welfare, 13*(3), 491-506.

Rosenstock, I. M. (1974). Historical origins of the Health Belief Model. *Health Education Monographs, 2,* 328-335.

Rosenstock, I. M. (1991). The Health Belief Model: Explaining health behavior through expectancies. In K. Glantz, F. M. Lewis, & B. K. Rimer (Eds.), *Health behavior and health education: Theory, research and practice* (pp. 39-62). San Francisco: Jossey-Bass.

Rosenstock, I. M., Strecher, U. J., & Becker, M. H. (1988). Social learning theory and the Health Belief Model. *Health Education Quarterly, 15*(20), 175-183.

Ross, H. S., & Mico, P. R. (1980). *Theory and practice in health education.* Mountain View, CA: Mayfield.

Rothman, J. (1970). Models of community organization. In F. M. Cox, J. L. Erlich, J. Rothman, & J. E. Tropman (Eds.), *Strategies of community organization: A book of readings* (pp. 3-26) Itasca, IL: F. E. Pecock Publishers.

Rotter, J. B. (1992). Cognates of personal control: Locus of control, self-efficacy, and explanatory style: Comment. *Applied and Preventive Psychology, 1*(2), 127-129.

Rubinson, L., & Alles, W. F. (1984). *Health education foundations for the future.* Propect Heights, IL: Moreland.

Rudd, R. E., & Walsh, D. C. (1993). Schools as healthful environments: prerequisite to comprehensive school health? *Preventive Medicine, 22*(4), 499-506.

Rumelhart, D. E., & Zipser, D. (1985). Feature discovery by competitive learning. *Cognitive Science, 9*(1), 75-112.

Sack, D. A. (1991). Use of oral rehydration therapy in the management of acute diarrhea. A practical guide. *Drugs, 41*(4), 566-573.

Sarason, S. B. (1984). *The psychological sense of community: Prospects for a community psychology.* San Francisco: Jossey-Bass.

147

Sarvela, P. D., & McDermott, R. J. (1993). *Health education evaluation and measurement: A practitioner's perspective.* Dubuque, IA: Brown & Benchmark.

Schall, E. (1994). School-based health education: What works? *American Journal of Preventive Medicine, 10*(Suppl. 3), 30-32.

Schiffman, L. G., & Kanuk, L. L. (1991). *Consumer behavior.* Englewood Cliffs, NJ: Prentice Hall.

Schwertfeger, R., Elder, J. P., Cooper, R., Lasatar, T. M., & Carleton, R. A. (1986). The use of telemarketing in the community-wide prevention of heart disease: The Pawtucket heart health program. *Journal of Community Health, 11*(3), 173-180.

Seaward, B. L. (1994). *Managing stress.* Boston: Jones & Barlette.

Seffrin, J. (1990). The comprehensive school health curriculum: Closing the gap between state of the art and state of the practice. *Journal of School Health, 60,* 151-156.

Selleck, C. S., Sirles, A. T., & Newman, K. D. (1989). Health promotion in the workplace. *American Association of Occupational Health Nurses Journal, 37*(10), 412-422.

Sellick, S., & Fitzsimmons, G. (1989). Biofeedback: An exercise in self-efficacy. *Medical Psychotherapy, an International Journal, 2,* 115-124.

Selye, H. (1976). *Stress in health and disease.* Woburn, MA: Butterworth.

Selye, H. (1978). *The stress of life.* New York: McGraw-Hill.

Seymour, H. (1984). Health education versus health promotion—A practitioner's view. *Health Education Journal, 43*(2&3), 37-38.

Setting the national agenda for injury control in the 1990s. (1992). *Morbidity and Mortality Weekly Report, 41,* 1-38.

Sheridan, C. L., & Perkins, A. (1992). Cross-validation of an inventory of stressors for teenagers. *Medical Psychotherapy, an International Journal, 5,* 103-108.

Shumaker, S. A., Schron, E. B., & Ockerie, J. K. (1990). *The handbook of health behavior change.* New York: Springer.

Simonds, S. K. (1978). The role of health education in public policy, ethics, and social justice. *Health Education Monographs Supplement, 6*(1), 18-27.

Sinha, D. P. (1992). Project lifestyle: Developing positive health lifestyles for school children in Antigua. *Journal of School Health, 62*(10), 449-453.

Sobel, D., & Hornbacher, F. (1973). *An everyday guide to your health.* New York: Grossman.

Society for Public Health Education. (1993). [Summary of Report of the AAHE/ SOPHE Joint Committee on Ethics]. (Copies can be obtained from SOPHE)

Solman, R., & Rosen, G. (1986). Bloom's six cognitive levels represent two levels of performance. *Educational Psychology, 6*(3), 243-263.

Statham, D. (1994). Working together in community care. *Health Visit, 67*(1), 16-18.

Steckler, A., & Dawson, L. (1982). The role of health education in public policy development. *Health Education Quarterly, 9*(4), 275-292.

Steckler, A., McLeroy, K. R., Goodman, R. M., Bird, S. T., & McCormick, L. (1992). Toward integrating qualitative and quantitative methods: An introduction. *Health Education Quarterly, 19*(1), 1-8.

Stokols, D. (1992). Establishing and maintaining healthy environments: Toward a social ecology of health promotion. *American Psychologist, 47,* 6-22.

Strecher, V., DeVellis, M., Becker, M., & Rosenstock, I. (1986). Self-efficacy and the Health Belief Model. *Health Education Quarterly, 13,* 73-92.

Strong, L. L., & Fiebert, M. S. (1987). Using paired comparisons to assess Maslow's hierarchy of needs. *Perceptual and Motor Skills, 64*(2), 492-494.

Sullivan, D. (1973). Model for comprehensive, systematic program development in health education. *Health Education Reports, 1*, 4-5.

Swisher, K. (1990). Cooperative learning and the education of American Indian/Alaskan Native students: A review of the literature and suggestions for implementation. *Journal of American Indian Education, 29*(2), 36-43.

Tannahill, A. (1985). What is health promotion? *Health Education Journal, 44*(4), 167-168.

Taras, H. L. (1994, Spring). School health clinics. *California Pediatrician*, pp. 31-33.

Taub, A., Kreuter, M., Parcel, G., & Vitello, E. (1987). Report of the AAHE/SOPHE Joint Committee on Ethics. *Health Education Quarterly, 14*(1), 79-90.

Tischler, H. L. (1993). *Introduction to sociology*. Fort Worth, TX: Harcourt.

Toohey, J. V., & Valenzuela, G. J. (1983). Values clarification as a technique for family planning education. *Journal of School Health, 53*(2), 121-125.

Tryon, W. W. (1976). A system of behavioral diagnosis. *Professional Psychology, 7*(4), 495-506.

Ulbrich, P. M., & Bradsher, J. E. (1993). Perceived support, help seeking, and adaptation to stress among older black and white women living alone. *Journal of Aging and Health, 5*(3), 365-386.

U.S. Preventive Services Task Force. (1989). *Guide to clinical preventive services: An assessment of the effectiveness of 169 interventions*. Baltimore: Williams & Wilkins.

U.S. Public Health Service. (1990). *Healthy people 2000: National health promotion and disease prevention objectives.*Washington, DC: U.S. Department of Health and Human Services.

U.S. Surgeon General. (1979). *Healthy people: The Surgeon General's report on health promotion and disease prevention*. Washington, DC: Government Printing Office.

Valente, C. M., Sobal, J., Muncie, H. L., Jr., Levine, D. M., & Antilitz, A. M. (1986). Health Promotion: Physicians' beliefs, attitudes, and practices. *American Journal of Preventive Medicine, 2*, 82-88.

Valente, T. W. (1993). Diffusion of innovations and policy decision-making. *Journal of Communication, 32*, 30-45.

Vincoli, J. W. (1993). *Basic guide to environmental compliance*. New York: Van Nostrand Reingold.

Vlisides, C. E., Eddy, J. P., & Mozie, D. (1994). Stress and stressors: Definition, identification and strategy for higher education constituents. *College Student Journal, 28*(1), 122-124.

Vogt, P. W. (1993). *Dictionary of statistics and methodology*. Newbury Park, CA: Sage.

Wagner, D. I. (1985). Future directions for health promotion program development in schools. *Special Services in the Schools, 1*(3), 125-134.

Wallack, L., Dorfman, L., Jernigan, D., & Themba, D. (1993). *Media advocacy and public health*. Newbury Park, CA: Sage.

Waller, J. V., & Goldman, L. (1993). Bringing comprehensive health education in the New York City public schools: A private-public success story. *Bulletin of New York Academy of Medicine, 70*(3), 171-187.

Wallerstein, N., & Bernstein, E. (1994). Introduction to community empowerment, participatory education, and health. *Health Education Quarterly, 21*(2), 141-148.

Wallston, B. S., Hoover-Dempsey, K. V., Brissie, J. S., & Rozee-Koker, P. (1989). Gate-keeping transactions: Women's resource acquisition and mental health in the workplace. *Psychology of Women Quarterly, 13*(2), 205-222.

Wankel, L. M., & Mummery, W. K. (1993). Using national survey data incorporating the theory of planned behavior: Implications for social marketing strategies in physical activity. *Journal of Applied Sport Psychology, 5*(2), 158-177.

Weiss, C. (1972). *Evaluation research: Methods for assessing program effectiveness.* Englewood Cliffs, NJ: Prentice Hall.

White, N. R. (1978). Ethnicity, culture and cultural pluralism. *Ethnic and Racial Studies, 1*(2), 139-153.

Whitehead, W. E., (1994). Assessing the effects of stress on physical symptoms. *Health Psychology, 13*(2), 99-102.

Williams, D. E., & Page, M. M. (1989). A multi-dimensional measure of Maslow's hierarchy of needs. *Journal of Research in Personality, 23*(2), 192-213.

Windsor, R., Baranowski, T., Clark, N., & Cutter, G. (1994). *Evaluation of health promotion, health education and disease prevention programs.* Mountain View, CA: Mayfield.

Windsor, R., Kronenfeld, J., Ory, M., & Kilgo, J. (1980). Method and design issues in evaluation of community health education programs: A case study in breast and cervical cancer. *Health Education Quarterly, 7*(3), 203-218.

Winett, R. A., King, A. C., & Altman, D. G. (1989). *Health psychology and public health: An integrative approach.* New York: Pergamon.

Winslow, C. E. A. (1920). The untilled field of public health. *Modern Medicine, 2,* 183.

Wooley, S. C., Blackwell, B., & Winget, C. (1978). A learning theory model of chronic illness behavior: Theory, treatment, and research. *Psychosomatic Medicine, 40*(5), 379-401.

Yates, S. (1994). The practice of school nursing: Integration with new models of health service delivery. *Journal of School Nursing, 10*(1), 10-19.

Zimmerman, B. J., & Rosenthal, T. L. (1974). Observational learning of "rules" governed behavior by children. *Psychological Bulletin, 81,* 29-42.

Zimmerman, R. S., & Olson, K. (1994). AIDS-related risk behavior and behavior change in a sexually active, heterosexual sample: A test of three models of prevention. *AIDS Education and Prevention, 6*(3), 189-204.

1990 Joint Committee on Health Education Terminology (1991). Report of the 1990 Joint Committee on Health Education Terminology. *Journal of Public Health Education, 22*(2), 97-107.

Suggested Readings

Abramson, J. H. (1979). *Survey methods in community medicine*. Edinburgh: Churchill Livingstone.

Aday, L. A. (1991). *Designing and conducting health surveys*. San Francisco: Jossey-Bass.

Ahijevych, K., & Bernhard, L. (1994). Health-promoting behaviors of African American women. *Nursing Research, 43*(2), 86-89.

Ajzen, I., & Madden, J. T. (1986). Prediction of goal directed behavior: Attitudes, intentions, and perceived behavioral control. *Journal of Experimental Social Psychology, 22,* 453-474.

Alexrod, M. (1975). Ten essentials for good qualitative research. *Marketing News, 10,* 10-11.

Allegrante, J. P., & Sloan, R. P. (1986). Ethical dilemmas in workplace health promotion. *Preventive Medicine, 15,* 313-320.

Arluke, A., Kennedy, L., & Kessler, R. C. (1979). Reexamining the sick role concept: An empirical assessment. *Journal of Health and Social Behavior, 20*(1), 30-36.

Ashton, J. (1990). Public health and primary care: Towards a common agenda. *Public Health, 104,* 387-398.

Baker, D., & Klein, R. (1991). Explaining outputs of primary health care: Population and practice factors. *British Medical Journal, 303*(6796), 225-229.

Bandura, A. (1977). *Social learning theory*. Englewood Cliffs, NJ: Prentice Hall.

Baranowski, T. (1981). Toward the definition of health and disease, wellness and illness. *Health Values, 5,* 246-256.

Barlett, E. E. (1982). Behavioral diagnosis: A practical approach to patient evaluation. *Patient Counseling and Health Education, 4,* 29-35.

Baronowski, J. (1992-1993). Beliefs as motivational influences at stages in behavior change. *International Quarterly of Community Health Education, 13*(1), 3-29.

Basch, C. E. (1987). Focus group interview: An underutilized research technique for improving theory and practice in health education. *Health Education Quarterly, 14,* 411-448.

Bauman, B. (1961). Diversities in conception of health and physical fitness. *Journal of Health and Human Behavior, 2,* 39-46.

Bauman, L. J., & Greenberg Adair, E. G. (1992). The use of ethnographic interviewing to inform questionnaire construction. *Health Education Quarterly, 19*(1), 9-23.

Public Health Promotion and Education

Becker, M. H., & Green, L. W. (1975). A family approach to compliance with clinical treatment. *International Journal of Health Education, 18,* 1-11.

Beilin, L. J. (1990). Diet and lifestyle in hypertension: Changing perspectives. *Cardiovascular Pharmacology, 16*(Suppl. 7), s62-s66.

Bellock, N. B., & Breslow, L. (1972). Relationship of physical health status and health practices. *Preventive Medicine, 1,* 409-421.

Bergan, J. R. (1980). The structural analysis of behavior: An alternative to the learning-hierarchy model. *Review of Educational Research, 50*(4), 625-646.

Berger, B., Hopp, J. W., & Raettig, V. (1975). Values clarification and the cardiac patient. *Health Education Monographs, 3*(2), 191-199.

Berger, P., & Neuhouse, R. (1977). *To empower people: The role of mediating structures in public policy.* Washington, DC: American Enterprise Institute for Public Policy Research.

Biersner, R. J. (1992). Assessing cognitive domain levels of instructional materials. *Perceptual and Motor Skills, 74*(3, pt. 1), 1010.

Birke, S. A., Eldermann, R. T., & Davis, P. E. (1990). An analysis of the abstinence violation effect in a sample of illicit drug users. *British Journal of Addiction, 85*(10), 1299-1307.

Bradley, R. H., Whiteside, L., Mundfrom, D. J., Casey, P. H., Kelleher, K. J., & Pope, S. K. (1994). Early indications of resilience and their relation to experiences in the home environments of low birthweight, premature children living in poverty. *Child Development, 65*(2), 346-360.

Breckon, D. J., Harvey, J. R., & Lancaster, R. B. (1994). *Community health education: Settings, roles and skills for the 21st century* (3rd ed.). Rockville, MD: Aspen.

Brick, P., & Roffman, D. M. (1993). "Abstinence, no buts" is simplistic. *Educational Leadership, 51*(3), 90-92.

Brieger, W. R., & Akpovi, S. U. (1982/1983). A health education approach to training village health workers. *International Quarterly of Community Health Education, 3*(2), 145-152.

Bruess, C. E. (Ed.). (1976). Professional preparation for the health educator. *Journal of School Health, 46*(7), 418-421.

Burns, D. D., & Nolen-Hoeksema, S. (1991). Coping styles, homework compliance, and the effectiveness of cognitive-behavioral therapy. *Journal of Consulting and Clinical Psychology, 59*(2), 305-311.

Carkenord, D. M., & Bullington, J. (1993). Bringing cognitive dissonance to the classroom. *Teaching of Psychology, 20*(1), 41-43.

Catalano, R., & Dooley, D. (1979). The economy as stressor: A sectorial analysis. *Review of Social Economy, 37,* 175-187.

Christianson, J. B., Lurie, N., Finch, M., Moscovice, I. S., & Hartley, D. (1992). Use of community-based mental health programs by HMOs: Evidence from a medicaid demonstration. *American Journal of Public Health, 82*(6), 790-795.

Chwee-Lye, C., & Giles, G. M. (1985). Behavior modification in the classroom: Some ethical reservations. *Education, 105*(4), 360-365.

Clark, N. M. (1978). Spanning the boundary between agency and community. *American Journal of Health Planning, 3*(4), 40-46.

Clark, N. M., Janz, N. K., Dodge, J. A., & Sharpe, P. A. (1992). Self-regulation of health behavior: The "Take PRIDE" program. *Health Education Quarterly, 19*(3), 341-354.

Clark, N. M., & Wolderufael, A. (1977). Community development through integration of services and education. *International Journal of Health Education, 20*(3), 189-199.

Clarke, K. R. (1983). The implications of developing a profession-wide code of ethics. *Health Education Quarterly, 10*(2), 120-125.

Clinefelter, J. S., & Knicker, C. R. (1980). Does values clarification go far enough? A report on classroom measurement of values. *Character Potential: A Record of Research, 9*(3), 155-165.

Coeling, H. V., & Wilcox, J. R. (1994). Steps to collaboration. *Nursing Administration Quarterly, 18*(4), 44-55.

Conrad, K. M., Riedel, J. E., & Gibbs, J. O. (1990). Effect of worksite health promotion programs on employee absenteeism. A comparative analysis. *American Association of Occupational Health Nurses Journal, 38*(12), 573-580.

Cooper, P. D. (1979). *Health care marketing: Issues and trends.* Germantown, MD: Aspen.

Corder, B. F., Whiteside, R., & Haizlip, T. (1986). Biofeedback, cognitive training and relaxation techniques as multimodal adjunct therapy for hospitalized adolescents. *Adolescence, 21*(82), 339-346.

Craigie, F. C., & Tan, S. Y. (1989). Changing resistant assumptions in Christian cognitive-behavioral therapy. *Journal of Psychology and Theology, 17*(2), 93-100.

Cross, H. D. (1994). An adolescent health and lifestyle guidance system. *Adolescence, 29*(114), 267-277.

Darr, K. (1991). *Ethics in health services management.* Baltimore: Health Professions Press.

Deeds, S., & Mullen, P. (Eds.). (1982). Managing health education in health maintenance organizations (Part 2). *Health Educational Quarterly, 9*(1), 3-95.

Deeds, S. G. (1992). *The health education specialist: Self study for professional competence.* Los Alamitos, CA: Loose Canon.

Delbecq, A. L., Van de Ven, A. H., & Gustafson, D. (1975). *Group techniques for program planning: A guide to nominal group and Delphi processes.* Glenview, IL: Scott, Foresman.

Deniston, O., & Rosenstock, I. (1973). The validity of non-experimental designs for evaluating health services. *Health Services Reports, 83*(7), 603-610.

Dignan, M. B., & Carr, P. A. (1992). *Program planning for health education and promotion.* Philadelphia: Lea & Febiger.

Duran, R. L., & Kelly, L. (1985). An investigation into the cognitive domain of communication competence. *Communication Research Reports, 2*(1), 112-119.

Dwyer, T., Viney, R., & Jones, M. (1991). Assessing school health education programs. *International Journal of Technology Assessment and Health Care, 7*(3), 286-295.

Eisen, M., Zellman, G. L., & McAlister, A. L. (1992). A health belief model social learning theory approach to adolescents' fertility control: Findings from a controlled field trial. *Health Education Quarterly, 19*(2), 249-262.

Elliott, C. H., Adams, R. L., & Hodge, G. K. (1992). Cognitive therapy: Possible strategies for optimizing outcome. *Psychiatric Annals, 22*(9), 459-463.

Eng, E., Salmon, M. E., & Mullan, F. (1992). Community empowerment: The critical base for primary health care. *Family and Community Health, 15*(1), 1-12.

Ferguson, E. (1993). Rotter's Locus of Control Scale: A ten-item two-factor model. *Psychological Reports, 73*(3, pt. 2), 1216-1278.

Ferrini, R., Edelstein, S., & Barrett-Connor, E. (1994). The association between health beliefs and health behavior change in older adults. *Preventive Medicine, 23*(1), 1-5.

Fisher, G. L., & Harrison, T. C. (1993). The school counselor's role in relapse prevention. *School Counselor, 41*(2), 120-125.

Fitzpatrick, J. L., & Gerard, K. (1993). Community attitude toward drug use: The need to assess community norms. *International Journal of the Addictions, 28*(10), 947-957.

Flay, B. R. (1987). Evaluation and development, dissemination and effectiveness of mass media health programming. *Health Education Research, 2*(2), 123-129.

Flinn, D., McMahon, T., & Collins, M. (1987). Health maintenance organizations and their implications for psychiatry. *Hospital Community Psychiatry, 38,* 255-263.

Flynn, B. C., Ray, D. W., & Rider, M. S. (1994). Empowering communities: Action research. *Health Education Quarterly, 21*(3), 395-405.

Fonnebo, V. (1994). The healthy Seventh-Day Adventist lifestyle: What is the Norwegian experience? *American Journal of Clinical Nutrition, 59*(Suppl. 5), 1124s-1129s.

Fowler, B. (1991). A health education program for inner city high school youths: Promoting positive health behaviors through intervention. *Association of Black Nursing Faculty in Higher Education Journal, 2*(3), 53-58.

Freda, M. C., Andersen, H. F., Damus, K., Poust, D., Brustman, L., & Merkatz, I. R. (1990). Lifestyle modification as an intervention for inner city women at high risk for preterm birth. *Journal of Advanced Nursing, 15*(3), 364-372.

French, B. N., Kurczynski, T. W., Weaver, M. T., & Pituch, M. J. (1992). Evaluation of the Health Belief Model and decision making regarding amniocentesis in women of advanced maternal age. *Health Education Quarterly, 19*(2), 177-186.

Friedman, R. A., & Podolny, J. (1992). Differentiation of boundary spanning roles: Labor negotiations and implications for role conflict. *Administrative Science Quarterly, 37*(1), 28-47.

Gallagher, H. G., & Phelan, D. M. (1992). Oral rehydration therapy: A Third World solution applied to intensive care. *Intensive Care Medicine, 18*(1), 53-55.

Garfinkel, A., Allen, L. Q., & Newharth-Pritchett, S. (1993). Foreign language for the gifted: Extending affective dimensions. *Roeper Review, 15*(4), 235-238.

Gilmore, G. D. (1977). Need assessment processes for community health education. *International Journal of Health Education, 20,* 164-173.

Glanz, K., Lewis, F. M., & Rimer, B. K. (Eds.). (1990). *Health behavior and health education: Theory, research and practice.* San Francisco: Jossey-Bass.

Gopaldas, T., Gujral, S., Mujoo, R., & Abbi, R. (1991). Child diarrhea: Oral rehydration therapy and rural mother. *Nutrition, 7*(5), 335-339.

Green, L., & Lewis, F. M. (1986). *Evaluation and measurement in health education.* Mountain View, CA: Mayfield.

Green, L. W. (1979). Health promotion policy and the placement of responsibility for personal health care. *Family and Community Health, 2,* 51-64.

Green, L. W. (1990). *Community health.* St. Louis, MO: Times Mirror/Mosby.

Grilo, C. M., & Shiffman, S. (1994). Longitudinal investigation of the abstinence violation effect in binge eaters. *Journal of Consulting and Clinical Psychology, 62*(3), 611-619.

Gruder, C. L., Mermelstein, R. J., Kirkendol, S., Hedeker, D., Wong, S. C., Schreckengost, J., Warnecke, R. B., Burzette, R., & Miller, T. Q. (1993). Effects of social support and relapse prevention training as adjuncts to a televised smoking cessation intervention. *Journal of Consulting and Clinical Psychology, 61*(1), 113-120.

Halpern, M. T. (1994). Effects of smoking characteristics on cognitive dissonance in current and former smokers. *Addictive Behaviors, 19*(2), 209-217.

Hanlon, J. J., & Pickett, G. E. (1984). *Public health administration and practice*. St. Louis, MO: C. V. Mosby.

Hochbaum, G. M., Sorenson, J. R., & Lorig, K. (1992). Theory in health education practice. *Health Education Quarterly, 19*(3), 295-313.

Hoppe, M. J., Wells, E. A., Wilsdon, A., Gilmore, M. R., & Morrison, D. M. (1994). Children's knowledge and beliefs about AIDS: Qualitative data from focus group interviews. *Health Education Quarterly, 2*(1), 117-126.

Horrine, F. (1966). Toward a philosophy of health education. *International Journal of Health Education, 9*(3), 106-112.

Housley, W. F., & Underwood, J. R. (1982). The use of values clarification in counselor education. *Counseling and Values, 26*(4), 228-235.

Iozzi, L. A. (1989). What research says to the educator. 2: Environmental education and the affective domain. *Journal of Environmental Education, 20*(4), 6-13.

Janz, N. K., & Becker, M. H. (1984). The Health Belief Model: A decade later. *Health Education Quarterly, 11*, 1-47.

Johnson, A. A., Knight, E. M., Edwards, C. H., Oyemade, U. J., Cole, O. J., Westney, O. E., Westney, L. S., Laryea, H., & Jones, S. (1994). Selected lifestyle practices in urban African-American women—Relationships to pregnancy outcome, dietary intakes and anthropometric measurements. *Journal of Nutrition, 124*(Suppl. 6), 963s-972s.

Kalnins, I., Mahon, S. M., & Casperson, D. S. (1994). Benefits of collaboration in continuing education: A partnership between a university provider and a nursing specialty organization. *Journal of Continuing Education in Nursing, 25*(4), 148-151.

Kasen, S., Vaughan, R. D., & Walter, H. J. (1992). Self-efficacy for AIDS prevention behaviors among tenth grade students. *Health Education Quarterly, 19*(2), 187-202.

Kashima, Y., Gallois, C., & McCamish, M. (1993). The theory of reasoned action and cooperative behavior: It takes two to use a condom. *British Journal of Social Psychology, 32*(3), 227-239.

Katz, P. P., & Showstack, J. A. (1990). Is it worth it? Evaluating the economic impact of worksite health promotion. *Occupational Medicine, 5*(4), 837-850.

Kee, K. N., & White, R. T. (1979). The equivalence of positive and negative methods of validating a learning hierarchy. *Contemporary Educational Psychology, 4*(3), 253-259.

Kirschenbaum, H. (1976). Clarifying values clarification: Some theoretical issues and a review of research. *Group and Organization Studies, 1*(1), 99-116.

Kirscht, J. P. (1974). The Health Belief Model and illness behavior. *Health Education Monographs, 2*, 387-408.

Knox, S. S. (1993). Perception of social support and blood pressure in young men. *Perceptual and Motor Skills, 77*(1), 132-134.

Kohler, C. L., Dolce, J. J., Manzella, B. A., Higgins, D., Brooks, C. M., Richards, J. M., & Bailey, W. C. (1993). Use of focus group methodology to develop an asthma self-management program useful for community-based medical practices. *Health Education Quarterly, 20*(3), 421-429.

Kothari, S. (1993). Effects of locus of control on anxiety and achievement-motivation. *Indian Journal of Psychometry and Education, 24*(2), 103-108.

Kotler, P. (1988). *Marketing management-analysis, planning and control*. Englewood Cliffs, NJ: Prentice Hall.

Kottke, J. L., & Schuster, D. H. (1990). Developing tests for measuring Bloom's learning outcomes. *Psychological Reports, 66*(1), 27-32.

Kraiger, K., Ford, J. K., & Salas, E. (1993). Application of cognitive, skill-based, and affective theories of learning outcomes to new methods of training evaluation. *Journal of Applied Psychology, 78*(2), 311-328.

Kreuter, M. W., & Green, L. W. (1978). Evaluation of school health education: Identifying purpose, keeping perspective. *Journal of School Health, 48*, 228-235.

Kronenfeld, J. J. (1993). *Controversial issues in health care policy.* Newbury Park, CA: Sage.

Langwell, K. M. (1990). Structure and performance of health maintenance organizations: A review. *Health Care Financial Review, 12*(1), 71-80.

Lewis, K. N. (1982). Values clarification: A critique. *Journal of Psychology and Christianity, 1*(1), 2-8.

Linstone, H. A., & Turoff, M. (1975). *The Delphi method: Techniques and applications.* Reading, MA: Addison-Wesley.

Maddux, J. E. (1993). Social cognitive models of health and exercise behavior: An introduction and review of conceptual issues. *Journal of Applied Sport Psychology, 5*(2), 116-140.

Mahon, N. E. (1994). Positive health practices and perceived health status in adolescents. *Clinical Nursing Research, 3*(2), 86-101.

Matteson, M. T., & Ivancevich, J. M. (1982). *Managing job stress and health.* New York: Free Press.

McAuley, E., & Shaffer, S. (1993). Affective responses to externally and personally controllable attributions. *Basic and Applied Social Psychology, 14*(4), 475-485.

McGinnis, J. M. (1993). The year 2000 initiative: Implications for comprehensive school health. *Preventive Medicine, 22*(4), 493-498.

Means, R. K. (1975). *Historical perspectives on school health.* Thorofare, NJ: Charles B Slack.

Mechanic, D. (1962). The concept of illness behavior. *Journal of Chronic Diseases, 15*, 189-194.

Mechanic, D. (1983). Adolescent health and illness behavior: Review of the literature and a new hypothesis for the study of stress. *Journal of Human Stress, 9*(2), 4-13.

Minkler, M. (1989). Health education, health promotion and the open society: An historical perspective. *Health Education Quarterly, 16*, 17-30.

Mooney, J. P., Burling, T. A., & Hartman, W. M. (1992). The abstinence violation effect and very low calorie diet success. *Addictive Behaviors, 17*(4), 319-324.

Morrison, E. M., & Luft, H. S. (1990). Health maintenance organization environments in the 1980s and beyond. *Health Care Financial Review, 12*(1), 81-90.

Moss, R. A. (1986). The role of learning history in current sick-role behavior and assertion. *Behavior Research and Therapy, 24*(6), 681-683.

Nader, P. R. (1990). The concept of "comprehensiveness" in the design and implementation of school health programs. *Journal of School Health, 60*(4), 133-137.

Narayanasamy, A. The application of performance indicators to nurse education (Part 2). *Nurse Education Today, 11*(5), 341-346.

Norman, P., & Conner, M. (1993). The role of social cognitive models in predicting attendance at health checks. *Psychology and Health, 8*(6), 447-462.

Nyswander, D. B. (1942). *Solving school health problems: The Astoria demonstration study.* New York: Commonwealth Fund.

Nyswander, D. C. (1956). Education for health: Some principles and their application. *California Health, 14,* 65-70.

O'Donnell, M. P. (1986). Definition of health promotion. *American Journal of Health Promotion, 1,* 4-5.

O'Donnell, M. P., & Harris, J. (1994). *Health promotion in the workplace* (2nd ed.). Albany, NY: Delmar.

Organista, K. C., Munoz, R. F., & Gonzalez, G. (1994). Cognitive-behavioral therapy for depression in low-income and minority medical outpatients: Description of a program and exploratory analyses. *Cognitive Therapy and Research, 18*(3), 241-259.

Parcel, G. S. (1976). Skills approach to education: A framework for integrating cognitive and affective learning. *Journal of School Health, 66,* 403-406.

Patrick, D. C., & Riggar, T. F. (1985). Organizational behavior management: Applications for program evaluation. *Journal of Rehabilitation Administration, 9*(3), 100-105.

Pender, N. J. (1990). Expressing health through lifestyle patterns. *Nursing Science Quarterly, 3,* 115-122.

Petosa, R., & Jackson, K. (1991). Using the Health Belief Model to predict safer sex intentions among adolescents. *Health Education Quarterly, 18*(4), 463-476.

Pollock, M. (1987). *Planning and implementing health education in schools.* Palo Alto, CA: Mayfield.

Rawson, R. A., Obert, J. L., & McCann, M. J. (1993). Relapse prevention strategies in outpatient substance abuse treatment. Special series: Psychological treatment of the addictions. *Psychology of Addictive Behaviors, 7*(2), 85-95.

Roberts, L. W., & Clifton, R. A. (1992). Measuring the cognitive domain of the quality of student life: An instrument for faculties of education. *Canadian Journal of Education, 17*(2), 176-191.

Rosen, G. (1958). *A history of public health.* New York: MD Publications.

Rotgers, F. (1985, June). Relapse prevention: Strategies for maintaining behavior change. *Carrier Foundation Letter (108),* 1-4.

Rousseau, C. (1993). Community empowerment: The alternative resources movement in Quebec. *Community Mental Health Journal, 29*(6), 535-546.

Rychlak, J., & Marceil, J. C. (1986). Task predication and affective learning style. *Journal of Social Behavior and Personality, 1*(4), 557-564.

Schlundt, D. G. (1988). Accuracy and reliability of nutrient intake estimates. *Journal of Nutrition, 118,* 1432-1435.

Shaw, M. E., & Wright, J. M. (1967). *Scales for measurement of attitudes.* New York: McGraw-Hill.

Somovar, L. A., & Porter, R. E. (1982). *Intercultural communication: A reader.* Belmont, CA: Wadsworth.

Sorensen, G. (1989). The relationships among teachers' self-disclosive statements, students' perceptions, and affective learning. *Communication Education, 38*(3), 259-276.

Stahl, N. N., & Stahl, R. J. (1991). We can agree after all—Consensus on critical thinking using the Delphi Technique. *Roeper Review, 14*(2), 79-88.

Steckler, A. B., Israel, B. A., Dawson, L., & Eng, E. (Eds.). (1993). Community health education. *Health Education Quarterly* (Supplement 1), S29-S47.

Stephens, R. S., et al. (1994). Testing the abstinence violation effect construct with marijuana cessation. *Addictive Behaviors, 19*(1), 23-32.

Stuart, K., Borland, R., McMurray, N. (1994). Self-efficacy, locus of control, and smoking cessation. *Addictive Behaviors, 19*(1), 1-12.

Suchman, E. A. (1967). *Evaluation research principles and practice in public service and social action programs.* New York: Russell Sage Foundation.

Tarver, S. G. (1986). Cognitive behavior modification, direct instruction and holistic approaches to the education of students with learning disabilities. *Journal of Learning Disabilities, 19*(6), 368-375.

Taylor, S. J., & Bogdan, R. (1984). *Introduction to qualitative research methods: The search for meanings.* New York: Wiley-Interscience.

Tiffany, S. T., & Cepeda-Benito, A. (1994). Long-term behavioral interventions: The key to successful smoking cessation programs. *Health Values: The Journal of Health Behavior, Education and Promotion, 18*(1), 54-61.

Titkow, A. (1983). Illness behavior and action: The patient-role. *Social Science and Medicine, 17*(10), 637-646.

U.S. Department of Health and Human Services, Office of the Assistant Secretary for Health. (1980). *Promoting health and preventing disease: Objectives for the nation.* Washington, DC: Government Printing Office.

Vitello, E. (1986). Ethical issues: Questions in search of answers. *Health Education, 17*(5), 39-42.

Walker, R. (1993). Modeling and guided practice as components within a comprehensive testicular self-examination educational program for high school males. *Journal of Health Education, 24*(3), 163-167.

Ward, T., Hudson, S. M., & Buliki, C. M. (1993). The abstinence violation effect in bulimia nervosa. *Addictive Behaviors, 18*(6), 672-680.

Weisbrod, R. R., Pirie, P. L., Bracht, N. F., & Elstun, P. (1991). Worksite health promotion in four Midwest cities. *Journal of Community Health, 16*(3), 169-177.

Welch, D. H., Luthans, F., & Sommer, S. M. (1993). Organizational behavior modification goes to Russia: Replicating an experimental analysis across cultures and tasks. *Journal of Organizational Behavior Management, 13*(2), 15-35.

White, R. T., & Gagne, R. M. (1978). Formative evaluation applied to a learning hierarchy. *Contemporary Educational Psychology, 3*(1), 87-94.

Whiting, S. (1994). A Delphi study to determine defining characteristics of interdependence and as potential nursing diagnoses. *Issues in Mental Health Nursing, 15*(1), 37-47.

Wilkin, D., Hallam, L., & Doggett, M. (1992). *Measures of need and outcome for primary health care.* New York: Oxford University Press.

Williams, T., & Jones, H. (1993). School health education in the European community. *Journal of School Health, 63*(3), 133-135.

Wilson, B. R., & Spivak, H. (1994). Violence prevention in schools and other community settings: The pediatrician as initiator, educator, collaborator, and advocate. *Pediatrics, 94*(4, pt. 2), 623-630.

Woodward, M., Bolton-Smith, C., & Tunstall Pedoe, H. (1994). Deficient health knowledge, diet, and other lifestyles in smokers: Is a multifactorial approach required? *Preventive Medicine, 23*(3), 354-361.

World Health Organization, Alma Ata. (1978). *Primary health care* (Health for All Series, no. 1). Geneva: Author.

Xiaojia, G. E., Conger, R. D., Lorenz, F. O., & Simons, R. L. (1994). Parents' stressful life events and adolescent depressed mood. *Journal of Health and Social Behavior, 35*(1), 28-44.

Zanga, J. R., & Oda, D. S. (1987). School health services. *Journal of School Health, 57,* 413-416.

About the Author

Naomi N. Modeste holds a Doctor of Public Health degree from Loma Linda University and is an Associate Professor in the Department of Health Promotion and Education, where she teaches Issues in Health Promotion and Education, and Health Education Program Administration. In addition to teaching, she coordinates the doctoral program in health education and the field practicum for the master of public health students. She is involved in research and has published several articles in refereed journals and in nonrefereed lay periodicals, as well as two Caribbean cookbooks. She has 18 years of experience as a health educator and administrator in the Caribbean and Latin America.